DEAD MEN DO
TELL TALES

DEAD MEN DO TELL TALES

✴

The Strange and Fascinating Cases of a Forensic Anthropologist

The hand of the Lord was upon me, and carried me out in the spirit of the Lord, and set me down in the midst of the valley, which was full of bones, and caused me to pass by them roundabout: and behold there were very many in the open valley; and lo, they were very dry. And he said to me, Son of man, can these bones live? And I answered, O Lord God, Thou knowest.

—Ezekiel 37:1–3.

To Margaret, Lisa and Cynthia, who never complained about the long hours I spent in the laboratory, or the bizarre stories I brought home. . . .
—W.R.M.

To Allison, Matthew and Noah, who know that the sun shines east, and the sun shines west. . . .
—M.C.B.

Table of Contents

DEAD MEN DO
TELL TALES

1

Every Day Is Halloween

I obtained leave to go down into the valley of death and gratify a reprehensible curiosity. . . . Death had put his sickle into this thicket and fire had gleaned the field. . . . The bodies [lay] half-buried in ashes; some in the unlovely looseness of attitude denoting sudden death by the bullet, but by far the greater number in postures of agony that told of the tormenting flame. Their clothing was half burnt away—their hair and beard entirely; the rain had come too late to save their nails. Some were swollen to double girth; others shriveled to manikins. According to degree of exposure, their faces were bloated and black or yellow and shrunken. The contraction of muscles which had given them claws for hands had cursed each countenance with a hideous grin. Faugh . . . !

—Ambrose Bierce, *What I Saw of Shiloh.*

I seldom have nightmares. When I do, they are usually flitting images of the everyday things I see on the job: crushed and perforated skulls, lopped-off limbs and severed heads, roasted and dissolving corpses, hanks of human hair and heaps of white bones—all in a day's work at my office, the C. A. Pound Human Identification Laboratory of the Florida Museum of Natural History at the University of Florida. Recently I dreamed I was in a faraway country, trying

1

on shoes, and the leather in the shoes was so improperly prepared that the laces and uppers were crawling with maggots. But there was a simple, ordinary explanation for this phantasm: one of my graduate students was raising maggots as part of a research project.

I have gazed on the face of death innumerable times, witnessed it in all its grim manifestations. Death has no power to freeze my heart, jangle my nerves or sway my reason. Death to me is no terror of the night but a daylit companion, a familiar condition, a process obedient to scientific laws and answerable to scientific inquiry.

For me, every day is Halloween. When you think of all the horror movies you have seen in your entire life, you are visualizing only a dim, dull fraction of what I have seen in actual fact. Our laboratory is primarily devoted to teaching physical anthropology to graduate students at the University of Florida, and is part of the Florida Museum of Natural History. Yet, thanks to the wording of the 1917 law establishing the museum, we often find ourselves investigating wrongful death, attempting to dispel the shadows surrounding murder and suicide. All too often in the past, under the old coroner system, the innocent have died unavenged, and malefactors have escaped unpunished, because investigators lacked the stomach, the knowledge, the experience and the perseverance to reach with both hands into the rotting remnants of some dreadful crime, rummage through the bones and grasp the pure gleaming nugget of truth that lies at the center of it all.

Truth is discoverable. Truth *wants* to be discovered. The men who murdered the Russian Tsar Nicholas II and his family and servants in 1918 imagined that their crime would remain hidden for all eternity, but scarce sixty years passed before these martyred bones rose up again into the light of day and bore witness against their Bolshevik assassins. I have seen the tiny, wisp-thin bones of a murdered infant stand up in court and crush a bold, hardened, adult killer, send him pale and penitent to the electric chair. A small fragment of a woman's skullcap, gnawed by alligators and found by accident at the bottom of a river, furnished enough evidence for me to help convict a hatchet murderer, two years after the fact.

2

The science of forensic anthropology, properly wielded, can resolve historical riddles and chase away bugbears that have bedeviled scholars for centuries. Reluctantly but carefully, I examined the skeletal remains of President Zachary Taylor, who died in 1850, and helped lay to rest persistent suspicions that he was the first of our presidents to be assassinated. The sword-nicked skull of the butchered Spanish conquistador, Francisco Pizarro, came within my field of inquiry, and I have held in my hands the bony orb that once enclosed vast dreams of gold, blood and empire. The gargoyle-like skull and skeleton of the Victorian-era "Elephant Man," Joseph Merrick, furnished me with pictures and impressions so poignant and vivid that I almost seemed to be conversing with the man himself.

But I do not seek out the illustrious dead to pay them court or borrow their fame. To me, the human skeleton unnamed and unfleshed is matter enough for marvel. The most fascinating case I ever had involved a modern, love-struck couple with very ordinary names: Meek and Jennings. It fell to me to extricate their bones, burned and crushed and commingled in thousands of fragments, from a single body bag, and put them back together again as best I could. When I was finished, after a year and a half's work, what I had was what lies deepest within all of us, at our center; that which is the last of us ever to be cut, burned, disassembled or dissolved; that which is strongest, hardest and least destructible about us; our firmest ally, our most trustworthy companion, our longest surviving remnant after we die: our skeleton.

I have often wondered whether I have a character flaw, to be so drawn to deathly things. I have always wanted to see the true facts of human existence, no matter how ugly. From a very early age I wanted to see life as it really was, not through the smudged windowpane of a newspaper or by means of the flickering picture of a movie newsreel. I wanted an uncensored view of reality. I did not want to know death from a neatly typed autopsy report, or from the body banked with flowers and surmounted by a stainless steel coffin lid at a funeral parlor. All my life I have been curious about death as it is, as it happens.

I was born in Dallas, Texas, on August 7, 1937. One of my grandfathers was a Methodist preacher, the other a saddle maker. My father was a banker who died when he was only forty, of cancer. I was just eleven. He was a man of strict morals who set a high premium on education. I grew up in a house filled with books and magazines such as *Collier's* and the *Saturday Evening Post*. The dictionary was one of the most used books in our library and reading was nearly as natural as breathing to me. I knew nine months before my father died that he was not going to recover, that the end was inevitable. This was a great sorrow to me; but in his last days my father said something that filled me with pride. He was giving some final instructions to my mother. He urged her to make sure that my brother, who was a splendid athlete, went to college. He did not mention me.

"What about Billy?" my mother asked him.

"Don't worry about Billy. He'll be all right," my father replied; and his deathbed faith in me has heartened me all my life.

One formative childhood event sticks out in my mind. It involved the great 1930s woman outlaw, Bonnie Parker, of *Bonnie and Clyde* fame. She crossed my path twice, even though she died before I was born. Bonnie was from Dallas and she first met Clyde Barrow, a native of Waco, in "Cement City," a rough part of Dallas near the Trinity River Bottoms, where she was working as a waitress. The pair went on to blaze their way across Texas and the Midwest and their legend was still fresh in Dallas when I was a boy. Our house was right across the street from the home of the chief deputy of the Dallas County Sheriff's Department.

One night this deputy, who was a friend of my father's, brought over the autopsy photographs of Bonnie Parker and Clyde Barrow. I was allowed to see them. They were the first autopsy photographs I had ever seen and they fascinated me. I was only about ten or eleven years old at the time. Far from being horrified, I was enthralled.

Years later, I happened to be wandering in a part of the cemetery where members of my family are buried in Dallas. I came upon a tombstone with this inscription:

AS THE FLOWERS ARE ALL MADE SWEETER BY
THE SUNSHINE AND THE DEW, SO THIS OLD
WORLD IS MADE BRIGHTER BY THE LIVES
OF FOLKS LIKE YOU

Above this poem were the words:

BONNIE PARKER
Oct. 1, 1910–May 23, 1934

I was astonished. The poem might have described a child or a sweetheart, instead of a cigar-smoking murderess who perished in a hail of bullets.

I later photographed this headstone and show the poem part in some of my lectures. The next slide shows the full epitaph, with the superscripted name: Bonnie Parker. In that moment in a Dallas graveyard it came to me that every person, from the most depraved serial killer to the most seraphic innocent, was likely loved by someone when each was alive. Victims and murderers alike are people. They may have followed their paths helplessly or of their own free will, but the paths led equally to the grave. All these people demand and deserve a dispassionate and caring analysis from investigators like myself. We can never forget that what we are doing is not just for the courts or for the general public. What we see on the table will have to be related to the families of victims and to the relatives of killers. Flowers and dew may seem far away from the microscopes and autopsy saws we employ, but they are still part of the picture. My wife's parents, my maternal grandparents and my father are all buried in that cemetery, in the same ground where Bonnie Parker lies.

I was brought up unreligiously, but with a set of hard, clear-cut moral values. Lies and laziness repel me more than the most putrefied corpse. If you wish to ponder the existence of the human soul or weigh whether there is life after death, you will have to seek elsewhere than in these pages. While I have seen consummate evil and its effects, I have never been overawed by it or attracted by the sleazy runways and approaches to it. The underside of life holds no personal fascination for me; nor have I ever been tempted to crawl into the gutter or stare through the sewer grate at the sordid practices of the living. I am not attracted to bars or nightclubs or bordellos, though I have hauled away and handled and examined the dead bodies of those who frequented them.

When people ask me how I ended up in forensic anthropology, I tell them it was a combination of good luck and bad character. I took my first anthropology course as an entering freshman at the University of Texas, purely by accident. Registration hours were nearly up. We freshmen always received the last appointments of the day. All the sections for introductory biology were filled up. My adviser suggested anthropology as an alternative.

"Fine. What's that?" I asked him.

"Try it. You may like it," he answered. So I found myself taking physical anthropology. I majored in English and minored in anthropology all through college and then, with just one semester left before graduation, switched my major to anthropology. One course required for the major was advanced physical anthropology, taught by a newcomer to the University of Texas, a man named Tom McKern.

It was McKern who, more than any other man save only my father, shaped and directed my life. McKern was . . . simply McKern. He was unique, a born teacher, a brilliant lecturer and a very charismatic personality. I soon learned that he had been born in Tonga, the son of an archaeologist, and had wide experience of foreign lands and far shores. He had worked at a laboratory in Tokyo, identifying the remains of American G.I.s killed at Iwo Jima in World War II, and later in Korea. Among the skeletons submitted to him for identification from the Iwo Jima battlefield was that of one of his closest friends, a man who had been best man at McKern's own wedding. McKern had seen extraordinary things, and there was a kind of glow about him. He fascinated and impressed every student who came into contact with him. He was what I would become: a forensic anthropologist.

That first day, McKern simply called the roll and dismissed the class. A few of us hung around afterward and chatted with him. He explained what forensic anthropology was, what it involved. He told us about testifying at trials, working with homicide cases. He said you could earn as much as a hundred dollars a day doing this extraordinarily fascinating work, if you testified in court. We were agog at this vast sum! The conversation lasted half an hour at most; but at the end of that half hour, when I walked out of that classroom, I knew what I wanted to do with my life.

Ever since I had turned eighteen I had been practically self-supporting. I paid my college expenses by working at a succession of odd jobs—*very* odd jobs. I was an attendant in a private sanitarium and had sometimes to restrain violent or delirious patients. I rode shotgun in an ambulance that belonged to a funeral home, and became proficient at throwing sheets with our home's name on them over the dead, mangled corpses of accident victims. The competition between rival funeral parlors for new business was fierce, and it made our work resemble some macabre rodeo, where the first cowboy who gets his rope over the steer wins, except that we were using sheets, not ropes, and we were flinging them over corpses, not steers.

Those were wild days, full of high-speed chases under Texas starlight. We would fly like bats from hell to the scene of an accident, risking our lives to pluck dead men off the asphalt first, ahead of the competition. We often took more chances getting there than the deceased took to die there. Our ambulance had a top speed of 105 mph, but we had a low-speed transmission. Our competitor's ambulance could do 110 mph but had a high-speed transmission. The difference in transmissions meant that our competitor could dust us on the flat straightaways out in open country, but we could show him our taillights in town.

We drove around at these breakneck speeds in the days before seat belts, and nothing we told the funeral parlor owner could persuade him to shell out for these safety restraints. This old man was a character. I remember him unfolding a whole set of membership cards for every conceivable organization in town. He belonged to all of them. As the cards riffled down to the tabletop he chuckled. "See these?" he said smugly. "Every one of them's a funeral!"

Then one night the owner happened to be riding in the ambulance himself and witnessed a particularly ghastly accident. A gravel truck had hit the rear fender of a car, spinning the car around and ejecting the seat-beltless driver like a child from a playground whirligig. The driver landed in the path of the truck, whose front wheels pulped his head. The sight of this atrociously mangled corpse softened even my boss's hard heart, and he equipped our ambulance with seat belts soon afterward.

I had been to funerals, but it was in those days that I saw my first dead body outside of a coffin. It happened my first night on the job. We were called to a house in Austin, where a woman was having severe chest pains. We found her wedged between her bed and the wall, wearing next to nothing. We hauled her out as gently as we could. She was still alive. We got her on a stretcher, put her aboard the ambulance and gave her oxygen on the way to the hospital. I was reassuring her all the way. Then, a few minutes after she was taken into the emergency room, as I looked on, she died.

Old Judge Watson—I have forgotten his first name—was called in to certify the death. The vertebrae in the judge's neck were fused together and he could no longer turn his head. So he would swivel his whole body, shoulders, head and all. He came in, looked down at the body, swiveled back and forth like a lighthouse for about half a minute, then croaked two words:

"Heart attack!"

That was all. The verdict was rendered. The authorities were finished with this woman. It was as though she had sunk beneath the surface of a dark sea. The stiff-necked old judge stumped out of the room, leaving us with the silent cadaver. Those two words were all the epitaph she got that night, and the sudden finality of it all impressed me greatly.

Certain scenes are engraved on my memory from those days. I remember the night we were called to the scene of a domestic dispute. A crippled husband had beaten his wife, using his crutch and the brass post from a four-poster bed. I remember another case in which a man got in a fight during which he was hit over the head with a large ketchup bottle. When we arrived the whole scene seemed to be weltering in red gore. I can stand the sight of blood, but the smell of it repels me. I did not think a human body could contain so much blood. In fact, it can't. A part of the sea of red was ketchup. The man survived and probably went on to other fights. I remember picking up a young man from an overturned car. He had a broken arm and moaned at me, asking where we were taking him. "The hospital," I said. Suddenly he began flailing away at me with both arms, broken and whole, trying to escape. It was all I could do to hold him down. It turned out he had stolen the car.

I saw terrible things during those nights, but I could not blink or turn away. My job depended on it. After a while it became a test of strength for me, to gaze unflinchingly at the dreadful aftermaths of accidents. Emergency room personnel deal with the same situations, but I would submit that the ER technicians see people after we ambulance men have tidied them up considerably. When we arrived at the scene, we were plunged into pure chaos. It was dark. Cars were overturned or on fire. Crowds were screaming. Police were yelling. Glass was broken. Smells of spilled fuel and roasted flesh were fresh. There is far more drama at the scene of an accident than there is in the emergency room afterward. At the hospital there are no shadows. Everything is clean and well lit and deodorized. Clean sheets and shiny instruments convey an atmosphere of relative calm and control. Already the horror is receding.

I saw my first autopsy when I was eighteen years old. Most of the autopsies in those days in Austin were done at the funeral homes, as they still are in many places. Pathologists would come in and do the cutting, weighing and photographing. Some of these specialists were very friendly and kind to us young laymen. They would let us stay and ask questions during the procedure. Gradually, I began to be exposed to decomposed bodies and severe trauma. Our funeral home had the contract to handle the remains of servicemen killed in military plane crashes. I saw bodies burned nearly to cinders. I saw the white, bloated bodies of young airmen recovered from the Gulf of Mexico. Many nights I had the eerie experience of sleeping in a room with burned bodies in bags all piled up and clearly visible just outside the screened door. It was at this period that I gradually developed my ability to work with bodies and manage to eat food. I remember having a chili-and-cheese hamburger in the autopsy room after an autopsy, looking at the burger carefully, then taking a bite, and then another, and another.

I saw tough policemen smoke cigars to keep the odors out of their nostrils. I remember the pathologist cutting through some medium-cooked soft tissue in a burned corpse while saying waggishly: "Well, I guess we don't want barbecued ribs for lunch today"—and seeing the police run from the room, green with nausea.

My life took on a strange, Jekyll-and-Hyde quality. By day, as an English literature undergraduate, I would contemplate the glories of Dickens, Trollope and Shakespeare. By night I would voyage into a world of dreadful pain and cruel misfortune, of flames and twisted steel, of bruisings, breakings and bleedings. I studied sonnets and suicides. I saw tragedies printed on paper and scrawled on asphalt. I dissected immortal poems from England and witnessed dead men and women cut carefully to pieces in Texas, under lamplight on stainless steel tables.

Then I was graduated. Margaret and I married one month before I took my B.A. at the University of Texas in January 1959. McKern encouraged me to go straight on to a Ph.D. in anthropology, skipping the master's degree. The University of Texas had no Ph.D. program in anthropology but McKern told me I could take courses elsewhere and he would supervise my progress personally. I decided, however, to work first for my master's degree.

It was useless. I flailed about in graduate school for a while, trying to make ends meet by moonlighting as a laboratory technician and grading exam papers. One summer I worked two jobs totaling forty-four hours a week, one of them as an athletic director in a school for retarded children, the other as a hospital orderly. At the same time I was attempting to take a full graduate course load. I was drained, exhausted after a year and a half. I was getting nowhere, it seemed. So as soon as Margaret won her degree in education I left school, went to Dallas and got a job with the Hartford Insurance Company as an investigator.

An old pathologist once told me: "When in doubt, think dirty. You'll be right ninety percent of the time." It was good advice, and I had many occasions to put it to good use while investigating insurance claims. Although I came to detest this job and the human vermin it brought me into contact with, in retrospect it was the best possible training for my later career as a forensic anthropologist. If any young man would care to find out in a hurry just how low his fellow human beings can sink, let him become an insurance claims adjuster. Whatever tender blossoms of altruism flowered in his innocent soul, these will be ripped out by the roots in six months flat; I guarantee it. At the same time, he will come face to face with some of the most vivid, brilliant, highly plausible fictions ever spun by human ingenuity. I know I did.

I shall not dwell on the tangled lies I had to unravel in those years. I learned to spot the people who specialize in falling down in front of vehicles. I learned about the "quick stop artists" who can brake their cars on a dime and cause rear-end collisions any time they like. I learned about physicians and chiropractors and the imaginative reports they would write about whiplash cases. I learned how reports were written charging that victims had suffered "permanent injury," even though there was not the slightest trace of any injuries and the doctors admitted as much. How could they then diagnose "permanent injury"? Easily: there might not be any permanent injuries *now;* but, they assured us, many "permanent injuries" develop *later* as a result of such accidents!

I had surreal talks with shyster attorneys, conversations that involved a complete suspension of belief on both sides. I would be talking to an attorney and would know he was lying and would know he *knew* I knew he was lying—and yet we had to talk on, grave-faced and sober, speaking in all seriousness, like two characters in a farce, fully cognizant of the fraud that choked the room like an invisible fog.

Nor was all the fault on the side of the victims. I saw insurance companies that wouldn't pay even though they were liable for accidents, because alert claims adjusters had swooped in early, beating the lawyers to the scene, and had obtained a statement from the victims that there were no injuries.

In those shabby days my esteem for the human race waned considerably. Toward the end, alarm bells would go off in my brain at the mere sound of those quavering, plaintive words: *"I just want what's due me."* All the lies and rigamarole instilled in me a real thirst for the truth, a realization that the truth is a valuable and rare commodity.

The skepticism of those days has stayed with me all my life and has made me a shrewder investigator than I might be otherwise. Some years later I caught a graduate student falsifying field notes in primate research in Africa. After I found he could not have been in the field, given his receipts and gasoline mileage, I fired him and sent him home. He said to me ruefully as I handed him his airline ticket: "You've always had a penchant for investigation."

At the time, however, I was miserable. I told Margaret that I wanted to go back to the ivory tower, back to the university. I wanted to get away from all the endless strife, controversy and dishonesty of the insurance business. I wrote my old teacher, Tom McKern, and asked if he thought I had the potential to become a forensic anthropologist, to make a career of it.

McKern wrote back and said, in essence: "Come." I went. In short order I earned my master's degree, put together my thesis on Caddoan Indian skeletons and had someone turn it in for me. By the time I learned I had won my master's degree, I was in Kenya, trapping baboons as part of a research project. I was an anthropologist, twenty-four years old.

No primate makes a good pet. That includes humans. We and our cousins—the gorillas, the chimpanzees, the monkeys, including the baboons—are a rather uncivilized lot, fiercely proud and independent, but at the same time treacherous, greedy, aggressive and cruel. I carry a deep scar on my right arm, where an old baboon bit me, lacerating my ulnar artery and coming very near to costing me a limb. I hold no grudge. It was a fair fight. In the eyes of the baboon I was certainly in the wrong. I had jabbed him with a tranquilizer in an effort to capture him alive in Kenya, to ship him to a research laboratory in America. In his position, I would have tried to kill me too.

My days in Africa marked me far more deeply than this hollow old wound in my arm shows. I caught malaria twice. I had to face down angry Masai tribesmen carrying spears. Wobble-kneed and drunk on pure adrenaline, I confronted charging Cape buffalo bent on trampling me to muddy paste, and shot them seconds before their horns got intimately acquainted with my chest. For sheer terror I recommend the Cape buffalo; no departmental chairperson or budget committee can begin to compare with this shaggy mass of bone, muscle and rage.

Kenya is forever glorious in my memory. In those magical times, thirty years ago, my wife and I were still discovering each other, truly building something together, amid the most exotic and beautiful surroundings imaginable. Both of our daughters were born in Nairobi.

My years in Kenya confirmed me in the path I had chosen. Africa poured forth gifts that I have always treasured, made me a better teacher, gave me a perspective that broadened and deepened my research. There is no greater living laboratory for anthropology on earth than the immensity of Africa, with its startling displays of nature, "red in tooth and claw," yet profoundly beautiful for all their savagery. What had been theoretical in my mind suddenly came to life before my eyes. I keep an articulated baboon skeleton on a shelf in my office, and it brings back memories of the Kenya and Tanzania I knew then: Kimana, where Hemingway camped and gazed at Kilimanjaro's snows; the blue Chyulu Hills, the Tsavo National Park, Lake Manyara where the lions lie lazily up in the trees, paws dangling from limbs; the magnificent Serengeti Plain, Lake Magadi, Lake Natron, the Ngurumani Escarpment.

I have tried to incorporate scenes from Africa into my lectures on anthropology and I think it has made them more interesting and down-to-earth. I can tell my students with eyewitness certainty that a lion will eat this but not that. I can set them straight about baboons, which are described in many textbooks as strict vegetarians, but which I have seen with my own eyes devouring hunks of freshly slaughtered baby antelope, chickens and other birds. Such lessons can't be learned in books. Africa tided me over during some very lean years in Academe, furnished me with ideas for research projects that ultimately helped me win tenure.

And it was all so magnificent: we breakfasted on mangoes and papayas. We saw plains of leaping oryxes, wildebeest and zebras, plains that scrolled out forever toward horizons of dust and rainstorms under purplish-blue skies. By night myriad stars shone, and in the limpid heavens the moonlight could be bright enough to read by. We had our clothes torn by "wait-a-bit" thorns, as they are called locally, and we roasted steaks of fresh-killed lesser kudu and impala at our campfires. At night the "bush babies," a wide-eyed species of lower primate also known as the galago, used to bounce on the tops of our tents as if they were trampolines, jumping up to catch bugs lured by the light of our encampment.

In those adventurous days I fought and fled from bush fires. I learned to fly, and piloted a plane over the Great Rift Valley, a vast geological feature that slices its way through East Africa. We traveled through the Ngorongoro Crater, a tremendous, extinct volcano whose rim encloses a tremendous ecosystem many hundreds of square miles in area, as green and gorgeous as some lost Eden. I took my wife and infant daughter for a visit to the mysterious Olduvai Gorge, and there we descended into the very deeps of time, where some of the earliest traces of man on earth have been found. The legendary Dr. Louis Leakey, who dug there for over thirty years and won a world-wide reputation as one of the giants of anthropology, hospitably treated us to lunch and tossed the salad with his own hands. I still have an old 8 mm home movie of the event, in which Leakey climbs the side of the gorge, scratching his bottom unselfconsciously, as any of the australopithecine protohumans might have done, in this same gorge, several million years earlier.

I owed my sojourn in Africa, which began in 1962, to the good offices of my teacher, Tom McKern. In those days an outfit called the Southwest Foundation for Research and Education, based in San Antonio, was interested in acquiring baboons. Baboons, it had been learned, have a peculiarity shared with humans: they can get atherosclerosis, or clogged arteries, from eating a normal diet. Any animal can get atherosclerosis if you force-feed it gobs of cholesterol, but the baboon can apparently get it eating the same things we do. This made baboons a valuable research animal, and the foundation was interested in acquiring specimens.

I served two tours at the foundation's primate research center in Kenya between 1962 and 1966. Altogether, we trapped and shipped hundreds of baboons back to America and their descendants are still in this country. It would not surprise me to learn that the baboon whose heart was transplanted into "Baby Fay" in a controversial and unsuccessful operation in 1992 in California was descended from baboon grandparents I trapped in Kenya.

I had seen baboons only in books and zoos before. Now I had to learn about them in the wild. I soon acquired the basics. Baboons run in troops numbering from about thirty to as many as two hundred individuals. There is considerable sexual dimorphism in baboons. Males and females differ markedly in size. Males weigh from about forty to sixty-five pounds. Females are much smaller and weigh from twenty to thirty pounds. Baboons are aggressive, but in most situations they are not a threat to humans unless they are trapped or if a young baboon is being threatened by a human within sight of its parents. They are fiercely protective of their young.

We trapped the animals with a variety of techniques. The most common type of trap was a cylinder of strong wire mesh, about five feet high, with more mesh welded to the top and bottom. This cylinder was fitted with a thirty-inch sliding door that could be raised and lowered in metal runners.

Inside the cylindrical trap we placed a small board shelf on two sticks, high up—too high for the baboon to stand outside and reach with his arm. On these shelves we placed our bait: maize. Baboons love maize. I have seen them running through maize fields in an orgy of gluttony, sticking an ear of maize under each arm, grabbing more ears, letting the first ears drop, replacing them with more ears, which fall when the next two ears are stolen. At the end of a row the baboon emerges with two ears of maize—and a whole trail of fallen and abandoned ears. They are the most improvident of thieves, forever stealing more than they can carry. I've known people who behaved in the same way, but that is another story.

Luring the baboons into the traps was a long task, requiring patience and cunning. First we scattered maize on the bare earth in a suitable clearing. Then we brought the traps in, set them up, and scattered maize around them. Then we scattered maize inside the traps, with the doors wired open. Then we put an ear of corn on the shelf, with the door still wired open. Finally, after the baboons were completely lulled into complacency by this glorious, never ending bounty of free food, we tied one end of a thread to the ear of maize and tied the other end to the falling door of the trap.

Bang! As soon as the baboon grabbed the ear of maize, the treacherous thread would break and down slammed the sliding door. When we arrived on the scene, there would be some very angry baboons gibbering and screaming and baring their fangs at us from inside the wire mesh traps. Amazing to relate, the creatures seldom had the wits to lift the door and escape. And they always ate the ear of maize clean, making the most of their time in captivity.

Now they were within our power, and now came the ticklish part: getting the baboons out of the traps and back to camp. We used a syringe crudely fitted to a hollow pipe to inject them with a tranquilizer. I later learned that this tranquilizer was an experimental drug, phencyclidine, now widely recognized as the main ingredient in the illicit drug known as "angel dust." It worked very well on the animals every time they had to be moved; but we noticed that after two or three doses they became violent and hard to handle whenever they saw us approaching with the pipe-syringe full of phencyclidine. I can only imagine that they did not have sweet dreams when under the influence of this drug. Certainly they came to hate it.

Our usual method was to hold the needle ready and approach the trap. Usually the caged baboon would jump away from the door and we would seize the instant to jab them in the thigh with the needle and push the plunger. The doses were done by rough guesstimate. We would look at a baboon and gauge the weight by visual inspection. In a few moments after the needle sank in, the beasts would get groggy. Then they would sway, totter and collapse on the cage of the floor. We waited a bit, then kicked the side of the cage to see if there was any reaction. Then came the moment of truth. I would open the door, grab the inert baboon firmly by the scruff of the neck and the base of the tail and haul the creature out of the trap. It is essential to act quickly and decisively: grab, grab, yank and hoist. If you move quickly and get the proper grip, it is very hard for the animal to turn its head and bite you.

All this I knew. All this I had done dozens of times. It was routine to me, second nature. Then one day, when I was hauling an old male baboon out of a trap, everything went horribly wrong. I had him by the neck and tail, there was no problem, everything was going according to plan. When I swung him up over the side of the pickup truck bed, his head swiveled around, so limply that it seemed to be lolling that way, merely because of gravity.

But in the next instant the cunning old fellow came to life and sank a razor-sharp canine tooth into my arm, a fang several inches long and sharp-edged along its inner curve. It went through my flesh like a stiletto. I was too astonished to feel much pain. I immediately fell to the ground on top of the animal and held his head as immobile as I could. If he managed to push my arm away with his powerful limbs, the tooth would rip clear through my arm muscles and arteries. I knew from experience that this is how a baboon fights, sinking its teeth into its enemy, then pushing the enemy away and letting the tooth tear through the flesh.

As I pinned the beast to the ground with the pierced arm, I beat him with my left fist on his zygomatic arch—the part of the skull near the cheekbone. It was some time before I could persuade him to open his mouth. I carefully unsheathed the long, bloody canine from my arm and disengaged it. The dripping-jawed old baboon was groggy enough to lie still on the ground now. I drove back to camp, the blood welling up from my wound in warm throbs. The ulnar artery had been nicked. I reached camp, leaped from the truck, ran for the first-aid kit and poured a surgical solution into the deep wound. It was approximately as soothing as napalm. I applied a pressure dressing to the wound and began dosing myself with erythromycin to fight infection. The nearest hospital was in Nairobi, a hundred and forty miles away, but before I could set out I had to wire all the trap doors open, in keeping with Kenyan game laws, so that no baboons could be caught in them and starve while we were away. I also had to give the old baboon who had wounded me another shot of phencyclidine. This time I erred on the side of caution, when it came to estimating the dosage.

I drove to Nairobi in a fog of pain. Every bump in the road reawakened my wounded arm. When I staggered into the hospital emergency room, the first thing the attendants said was: "Look at his color. He's in shock." And I remember thinking blurrily: "My God, I'm in shock." My arm looked as if it belonged to Popeye the Sailor, it was so puffed up with blood from the leaking ulnar artery.

And so began an uncomfortable convalescence. Despite the erythromycin I'd administered back at the camp, *E. coli* bacteria spread and proliferated in the wound. The swollen arm stank so much it seemed to belong not to me but to a corpse. I slept with the limb outstretched, trying to get as far from it as I could. For a while the arm looked as if it might have to be amputated. But with time, and many soakings in Epsom salts, the swelling gradually abated and the wound was purged clean. It was a near-run thing.

Far from being soured on Kenya because of my wound, I became fonder of it than ever, as if the country had entered my heart through a hole in my arm. Phrases and fragments of Swahili recur to my mind at odd moments and, even though they are tattered now with the passage of time, the bits I remember still have a beautiful, vital ring in my ears. I remember how a can opener was called a *tinikata,* a wagon a *gari,* and a train a "smoke wagon," a *gari la moshi.* I still use some Swahili phrases today because they are wonderfully descriptive. A barbarian, an uncivilized person, is a *shenzi.* An utter fiasco is a *shauri.* One of the medical examiners in Florida also lived in Kenya for a time and it is a great pleasure to greet him with a hearty *"Jambo, bwana* [Good day, sir]!"—and to hear the same in return.

Isaac Newton once complimented his forerunners in science, whose research enabled him to formulate the first laws of physics. "If I have seen further," Newton said, "it is because I have stood upon the shoulders of giants." In my case, it has been the shoulders of baboons, but I am nonetheless grateful.

Talkative Skulls

People begin to see that something more goes to the composition of a fine murder than two blockheads to kill and be killed—a knife—a purse—and a dark lane. Design, gentlemen, grouping, light and shade, poetry, sentiment, are now deemed indispensable to attempts of this nature.

—Thomas De Quincey, *On Murder Considered as One of the Fine Arts*

One of Sir Arthur Conan Doyle's most amusing short stories, "Crabbe's Practice," deals with the desperate attempts of a young doctor to set himself up in the world and acquire patients. Hoping to burnish his academic reputation, he publishes a deep and erudite paper in a medical journal, with the bizarre title, "Curious Development of a Discopherous Bone in the Stomach of a Duck." Later he confesses to a friend that the paper was a fraud. While dining on roast duck, the young doctor discovered that the fowl had swallowed an ivory domino, and he had turned the experience into a research paper. "Discopherous" is just a Greek term for "circle-bearing," and refers to the circular dots on a domino.

Conan Doyle was a doctor himself and knew whereof he spoke. Anyone who works in science knows the dull desperation and sharp anxiety of the early days in one's career. Few of us do not look back on those pinched, scraping times without a secret shudder, followed by a pang of relief that they are past. The miserable pay and financial woes; the long nights of study and the battles against sleep; the frightful hurdles of examinations; the climactic defense of one's doctoral dissertation; the hissing, malignant envy that is the curse of university life at all times and in all places; the constant struggle to get published, to win tenure, to carve out a niche and be recognized in one's field—all these torments are well known in Academe, and have been known to drive some people mad, even to suicide. Some people. Not me.

My early experiences riding shotgun in the funeral parlor's ambulance in Texas had shown me a side of life no book could teach. These dreadful sights gave me a certain balance, along with reserves of strength that I could call on in the ordinary trials of life at the university. When you have seen bodies burned to cinders in fires, or pummeled to jelly under a truckload of bricks, or reduced to empty skins whose bones have been squeezed from them by the terrific force of plane crashes, then the bumps and bogies of academic life hold few terrors for you. "It could be worse," you tell yourself; and when worse is the thing you saw lying dead in a highway culvert scarcely twelve hours earlier, you know you are telling the truth.

The first time I was asked for my considered opinion about a skull came when I was still in graduate school, still working under Tom McKern in his laboratory. It was a watershed moment for me, because for the first time McKern was treating me—I will not say as an equal, but very nearly as a colleague whose independent opinion he valued.

On that morning when I came into the laboratory McKern presented me with a cranium, a skull without the lower jaw. It had been found in Lake Travis near Austin with a fishing line tied around the zygomatic arch, the cheekbone. The other end of the fishing line was tied to a large rock.

As I handled the still damp cranium, my attention was drawn to the palate. More than anything else, the shape of that palate struck me. It stood out, to my eyes, in a very unusual way. Looking at it, I was racked by doubts. I felt very insecure because obviously McKern was going to judge me on my response. More than that, I was insecure because I was about to give him an answer I felt was intrinsically improbable. At last I summoned up my courage and spoke:

"I think it's Mongoloid, probably Japanese," I said. McKern looked at me for a long moment. Then at last he said: "That's what I think too."

Whatever pride I felt was immediately dampened by McKern, who went on to point out all the other things I had missed. With the sure touch of a true master of forensic anthropology, he demonstrated one detail after another, details which I had seen but had not observed. At such times McKern was truly dazzling and I shall never forget those lucid, decisive moments in which he practically made that old skull speak.

I had *not* observed that some of the teeth had been glued into their sockets. I had *not* observed the scorching on the outer cranial vault. I had *not* observed the very simple fact that the skull had been attached to a fishing line tightly tied to its zygomatic arch, which meant that it was dry, unfleshed bone to start with, when it was plunged into the lake.

After McKern had pointed out all these things, the answer became clear. The skull before us was almost certainly a World War II trophy skull that some serviceman brought back from the Pacific Theater. The scorching had occurred during battle, perhaps by the action of flamethrowers or as the result of a fiery plane crash. The teeth had fallen out as the skull dried out and had been glued back in. Finally, either the serviceman himself had sickened of his gruesome relic, or he had died and his heirs wanted to get rid of the thing. But how to dispose of it? If they put it in the garbage it might be found. Burning it was too much trouble. Burying it would be bothersome and might leave traces. Best to throw it in the lake! Tie a rock to it for good measure! And so the skull went overboard, bubbling down into the depths of Lake Travis, only to be found again by the purest chance.

I am certain that, somewhere in Japan today, there is a family wondering what became of an uncle, a father, a long-lost relative who marched off to war more than half a century ago. They will never know. And the Japanese man whose skull this was, how could he have dreamed that, after great and fiery battles in the middle of the vast Pacific, the bony vessel enclosing his dreaming brain was destined to end up tied to a rock and drowned in a cool American lake, then fished up onto a bright laboratory table at the University of Texas?

The television show "Quincy" has caused me no end of vexation and amusement. When people learn that I am a forensic anthropologist, the first thing they usually say is: "Oh, like Quincy?" Quincy was a medical examiner whose whole career was one long string of dramatic successes. Born under a lucky star, Quincy solved his cases within hours or days. If Quincy had a problem, he telephoned his brilliant assistant, Sam, back at the lab, and Sam had the answer for him in seconds. Sam! How I envied Quincy his faithful and unerring Sam! Any one of us could shine like the morning star if we only had a Sam working for us. In one episode Quincy and Sam actually determined the hair color of a skeleton by examining its femur—a complete scientific impossibility. A bunch of us forensic anthropologists later cornered the technical advisor of this episode at the annual convention of the American Academy of Forensic Scientists. Up against the wall, needled and jabbed by our merciless questions over this hair-color episode, he finally admitted that he had taken "dramatic license" to "move the plot forward."

I am not Quincy. The difference between forensic pathologists and forensic anthropologists is quite simple. Pathologists have medical degrees. They are doctors who have received residency training in pathology. If they are fortunate, they also have some training in courtroom procedures. All the medical examiners in the state of

Florida are forensic pathologists with medical degrees. In some states they may also serve as county coroners, legally determining the cause of death. But in others, the coroner may have no medical background at all; he may simply be a local person with a reputation for shrewdness and honesty. I have known coroners who were filling station owners, or funeral parlor directors, or even furniture salesmen. Why furniture salesmen? Because in the old days these merchants stocked coffins in their shops.

A forensic anthropologist is not a medical doctor, though he has a Ph.D. and has studied anthropology in college. We specialize in the human skeletal system, its changes through life, its changes across many lifetimes, and its variations around the world. We are part of the larger field of physical anthropology, or biological anthropology as it is known today, which is concerned overall with the human body and all its variations. My specialty, physical anthropology, is distinct from other fields, such as cultural anthropology and archaeology. The cultural anthropologists are the ones who go out and study the exotic tribes, the *"fluttered folk and wild,"* as the poet Rudyard Kipling called them. The archaeologists look for tools and other evidence of ancient and recent man in the folds and hollows of Asia, Africa and Europe.

My field of expertise is the human skeleton. Though some pathologists insist on doing their own skeletal examinations along with autopsies, I can confidently say that there are very few cases in which a forensic anthropologist—someone like me—could not add a great deal of useful information to what a pathologist can discover. I have had pathologists exclaim frankly in my hearing, when confronted with a skeleton: "Gee, I'm not used to looking at these without the meat on them!"

But long and lean were the years from the time I entered graduate school, in 1959, to the time I got my first case, in 1972. There was a spot of work from time to time in McKern's lab. There were occasional formal examinations of skeletons in Africa. But apart from these cases, the annals of my professional life in this period are rather parched and poor.

When I open my filing cabinets the gaunt memories of those starveling years come back to me vividly. In 1972 I had but a single case. In 1973 hope blazed up like a bonfire: a scatter of buried bodies was found less than a quarter of a mile away from where I live in Gainesville. These remains turned up when new utility lines were being laid, and for a while it was feared that we were dealing with the grisly spoils left by a serial killer. The former owner of the house in whose backyard these bodies came to light was an attorney who had committed suicide years earlier. All sorts of wild theories were floating about.

The police asked me and three university archaeologists to investigate. We all piled into a van and drove to the site. Within a few hours we had turned up casket hardware, nails, screws, etc., that indicated we were dealing with nothing more sinister than an early twentieth-century graveyard. The whole thing was a fiasco, a false alarm.

In 1974, I had two cases. In 1975, two more cases; in 1976, two cases; in 1977, three cases; in 1978—twelve cases! And from then on things began to snowball.

When the Florida Museum of Natural History was endowed by the state legislature in 1917 as the Florida State Museum, one of its functions, as spelled out in the original wording of the law, was that the museum would provide assistance to the state in "identifying specimens." I doubt the original framers of the law imagined that among those "specimens" would be human remains, still less that those remains would be the ghastly leavings of murderers and maniacs. But over the years I have tried to do my part to repay the generosity and vision of those state legislators of long ago. My first opportunity to do so—my first case—came in April 1972, when a Washington County sheriff's deputy brought me a peat-encrusted skeleton that had been found in the woods and asked me to analyze it.

The skeleton had been found in a swamp near Chipley. There was no name, no identifying information accompanying it at all. I took the skeleton down to the steam tables at the end of my laboratory in the basement of the anthropology department and started cleaning away the vegetable matter. Meanwhile a class nearby broke for coffee and the professor brought his pupils over to see what I was doing. This professor was a bit of a twit. He said to the students, very jocularly: "You see, science has its uses in the real world." I was irritated at his condescension but concealed it. I invited the students to have a look at the skeleton. They crowded over.

"Here are his socks," I said. "And you can see the feet are still in the socks."

At that point the twit vanished from the scene and so did most of his fainthearted students. I learned the power of cold reality, how it acts like a fly whisk to chase idle minds away; and I admired those students who stayed behind.

You always have a fondness for your first cases, and I found this skeleton very interesting. Under analysis, it turned out to be that of a toothless elderly man with a lot of union or fusion of bones in his back, due to old age. The really fascinating thing was that he had a large opening where one ear would have been on the skull. It was all hollowed out and eaten away. Obviously he had been deaf in that ear. But there was more: a penetration from this area up through the thin bones above, which meant that this perforation went into the cranial vault, the brain case. Finally, along the inner surface of that brain case you could see pitting, where an infection had eroded the bone during life.

I went to the University of Florida Medical School library, researched the problem and found abundant literature that described the condition. It was a middle ear infection. Such an infection, if not treated, will cause hearing loss and excavation of the bony surface in the area. Sometimes this gnawing will penetrate the brain case, leading to infection that would cause disorientation, nerve problems and death. In its earlier stages the infection produces a dripping exudation from the ear that would be foul-smelling.

Armed with this information, I asked the sheriff if there were any local people who fit this description. It turned out there was a man, a retired farm laborer living on Social Security, who was well known in the vicinity and who had been missing for two years. His name—there is no need to give his name; he was subsequently identified beyond doubt. Toward the end of his life a foul odor hung about him, so oppressive that people shunned him. From his tottering gait, he also seemed to have motor nerve problems. People thought he had suffered a stroke and was partially paralyzed. Neighbors and acquaintances confirmed that he seemed increasingly disoriented toward the end of his days. Finally he wandered off and disappeared, not to be seen again until the skeleton was retrieved from the swamp.

But the skeletal remains that had moldered for two years in the wild could still speak to me. The perforated skull with the pitted brain case yielded up information that agreed very well with reports of the man in life. It could even describe to me the last hours of the unfortunate farmhand, shunned and alone, stumbling into the swamp in pain, his brain swarming with infectious invaders that gnawed away at his balance, his reason and the very bone that encased his brain.

I handed the skeleton back over to the sheriff's office, together with my findings. Once, long afterward, I was traveling through Chipley and stopped in at the sheriff's office to ask about the final disposition of the case. The deputies told me that the coroner had ruled the farmhand had been clearly identified and had died a natural death.

In 1974, almost in desperation, an investigator with the Eighth Judicial Circuit of the state attorney's office brought me a portion of a cranium just a few days before a trial was going to begin. This skullcap had been found by scuba divers near a bridge over the Santa Fe River, the northern boundary of Alachua County, on September 1, 1974, about seventy yards away from a spot where, nearly two years previously, the remains of a headless, handless female body had been found. This headless trunk was identified by certain surgical scars, which were still visible on the torso, as belonging to a Union County woman who had been abducted on August 23, just nine days earlier. At the same time she vanished, a farm laborer named Raymond Stone also disappeared. Stone was later captured in Missouri and, under questioning by police, confessed to killing the woman. Later, however, he retracted his confession.

There was no evidence of trauma or foul play to be found on the woman's torso. The local medical examiner looked at the body and concluded that the head had been gnawed off and carried away by alligators after the woman's death. Then the divers found the skull-cap.

This medical examiner—there is no need to name him—was an extremely arrogant individual, supremely self-assured, who airily told the sheriff's investigators, when the skullcap was found, that there was "nothing you could tell from an old, dry bone." He refused to do any analysis at all.

Almost apologetically, the state attorney's investigators approached me with the skull fragment and asked me if I could tell them anything about it. I analyzed the remains and, working against the clock because the trial was imminent, made a report in just seventy-two hours. I said this skullcap belonged to an adult white female. She was mature but had not yet reached middle age. The shape of the upper margins of the orbits (eye openings), the smooth, high forehead and the muscle attachment markings were all consistent with a female. Age could only be deduced from the cranial sutures, the "stitches" where the various plates of our skull are joined. This is a notoriously unreliable technique, but in this case it was all I had to go by; therefore my age estimate was carefully vague.

I told the deputies that the woman had been struck at least twice by a weapon that had a hammerlike aspect to it. One of the fractures was a round penetration of the frontal bone, which clearly showed the circular mark of the hammer. A small portion of bone was broken at the edge but hinged downward, indicating that the bone was fresh and elastic when the injury took place. Fracture lines radiated out from this penetration. There was another, second injury, that consisted of a depressed skull fracture of the outer layer of the cranial vault. Here the outer layer had been mashed down, but again you could see clearly the flat, circular striking surface of the hammer head. A depressed skull fracture of this type is also an indication that the bone was still fresh and elastic when the blows were struck. The skull resembles an eggshell that has been cracked but not quite broken through.

When the investigators first came to me they told me in strictest confidence that they had a suspect who was already in custody; that this suspect had confessed to murdering the woman whose headless body had been found in the Santa Fe River in 1972; but that this same suspect had later retracted his confession. The suspect, they told me, had confessed that he had used a hatchet to commit the murder—a hatchet, not a hammer.

The trial took place at Lake Butler, Union County. I remember waiting for hours to testify, sitting on a wooden staircase, which was the only available place for witnesses to wait. It was the first time I testified as an expert witness in a murder case, and it went awkwardly. The prosecutor tried to ask me very controlled, step-by-step questions, instead of simply asking me: "What did you find?" For my part, I tried to treat the jury as if they were a class of undergraduates, to testify as if I were teaching, and that is a mistake too. I even made an attempt at humor, the way a teacher does when he is trying to keep the class's attention. Whatever the jest was, it fell terribly flat and in that embarrassing instant there was seared into me a lesson I have never forgotten since: a courtroom is not a classroom.

The great riddle of the trial, the hammerlike blows that had apparently been made by a hatchet, was eventually solved. I was just one of many witnesses called, and I was not privy to the other evidence in the case until after the trial. Then I learned that the hatchet the defendant had used was a carpenter's hatchet, with a blade on one side of the head and a hammer on the other. Even so, I was puzzled: why would he use the hammer side and not the hatchet side to kill? I have learned the answer since. Hammer blows do not spatter blood as much as ax blows do. It is a question of economy and neatness.

I shall never forget Raymond Stone's appearance when I first laid eyes on him in court. He was a very, very small, thin man who was going bald. He wore a light blue cardigan sweater—I have since learned it is an old courtroom ploy to dress defendants in loose-fitting, baggy clothes. It makes them look smaller and less threatening. I remember thinking that Stone looked like my barber in Gainesville. How could someone so meek and kindly-looking do what Stone was accused of doing? How could he have bludgeoned an innocent woman to death and flung her body from a bridge?

At the trial it came out that, at the time of the murder in 1972, Stone had been working as a hired hand on a farm owned by the victim and her husband. The murder probably had something to do with a spurned sexual advance on Stone's part. He had propositioned his boss's wife and been refused; enraged, he had killed her. Stone was convicted and Judge John J. Crews sentenced him to death. At his sentencing, Stone threatened to "raise hell" and tried to spit on the judge. But this frail-looking, malignant man is still alive as I write these lines, and on February 7, 1994, his death sentence was commuted to life imprisonment. Stone's lawyers were able to win a resentencing for him because evidence about his background and unhappy childhood was not heard by the jury at his original trial. Stone grew up in a Missouri garbage dump, sleeping in an abandoned truck. His father murdered Stone's mother when the boy was nine, and allegedly beat the boy and sexually abused him. Stone had spent much of his life in jails and mental hospitals. A higher court ruled that the jury ought to have been told all this before it recommended the death penalty in Stone's case.

Despite the resentencing, it is thought unlikely Stone will ever be paroled. He has survived three heart attacks and has undergone bypass surgery in prison. I have also since learned from prison officials that Stone is something of a pariah in prison. Even when he was on Death Row, the other condemned men regarded him as a human rattlesnake.

The skullcap in the Stone case was a victory, not so much for me as for the science of forensic anthropology in Florida. It was the last link in the chain of evidence that connected Stone with his victim.

The sutures and shape established the age and sex of the owner; the trauma marks established the shape and type of the weapon. I was able to join the skullcap to the body that had been found two years earlier, and the skullcap was the most eloquent, damning piece of evidence in the case. This victory was owed to good luck, hard work and the mercy of the alligators who gnawed the victim's head away from her body. In the end, it was the alligators of the Santa Fe River who left this crucial fragment of bone to be retrieved by the scuba divers and to tell its tale in court.

The Stone case had an unexpected sequel about three years ago when the daughters of the deceased woman asked to see the records of the trial, in order to learn more about the death of their mother. The young ladies were received with courtesy at the Lake Butler courthouse, but when the filing cabinet was opened a ghastly sight awaited them: there, still in the drawer, was their mother's bludgeoned skullcap!

The two were understandably upset and begged that the fragment be released to them immediately for proper burial. It was a ticklish question, since Stone was still alive and going through the endless appeal process that accompanies any death sentence. The current Alachua County medical examiner and I discussed the case and concluded, since we had abundant photographs that could be used in the event of any retrial, that there was no impediment to the skullcap's release. So the two daughters bore away the last bit of their unhappy mother's head and buried it.

"Bolts of Bones"

O Who shall, from this Dungeon, raise
A Soul enslav'd so many wayes?
With bolts of Bones, that fetter'd stands
In Feet; and manacled in Hands
Here blinded with an Eye; and there
Deaf with the drumming of an Ear.
A Soul hung up, as 'twere in Chains
Of Nerves, and Arteries and Veins
Tortur'd besides each other part
In a vain Head and double Heart . . .

—Andrew Marvell,
  A Dialogue Between the
  Soul and Body

The unwary visitor to the C. A. Pound Human Identification
Laboratory might be pardoned an involuntary gasp of shock. Inside
this unobtrusive building, hidden in a grove of thick bamboo off
Radio Road in Gainesville, death grins at you from every angle,
massed, multiplied and compressed with terrific force within a very
narrow compass. My laboratory room itself is not large, perhaps the
size of two living rooms; but on its tables, in its shelved boxes, in its

labeled specimen jars and phials, are the full and partial skeletons of a silent throng of people, all awaiting identification, or their day in court, at the trials of their killers. It is a fleshless village of the dead, dry and silent save for the soft whirr of a dehumidifier under a table.

But this finality is an illusion. Just as in the book of Ezekiel, the dry bones knit themselves back together, are covered anew with flesh, draw breath and at last stand forth as a living host of human beings, so the remains in this room have begun a second life, a life after death. They are speaking secrets to me and to my students, yielding up hidden information, furnishing ideas and evidence to the world of the living. The truth is germinating in them, sprouting up vividly. Remains such as these have established innocence or guilt. They have pointed the way to the electric chair.

Here lie bones burned and boiled, drowned and desiccated; bones that once lay buried, long forgotten, are now summoned back suddenly into the light of day; bones of martyred innocents, and bones of double-dyed murderers, all lying side by side, equal and silent beneath the impartial eye of science. We have few living visitors, and those who are admitted must show they have good reason to enter. But the dead are welcomed, and we show them every courtesy. As you stare about, you may see some cranial vaults showing clear bullet holes, dark circles where death entered and overtook the owners, extinguishing life as a puff of air blows out a candle. Against a far wall there hangs a translucent death mask, silhouetted on film against the milky-bright shine of an x-ray light table. It is the radiograph of a broken skull, showing a spangling of lead particles shining like lethal dew, sprinkled throughout the braincase. It belongs to a gunshot victim.

On most days the air in my laboratory is cool, chalky, clean-smelling, with a hint of fresh, wet earth. On those days, no reek of decay pollutes the atmosphere. In one corner you may see a young graduate student tweezering his way slowly through a heap of clay clods, separating out the tumbled teeth and vertebrae of an apparent suicide, years old. Hanks of human hair from plane crash victims are nearby, shampooed and shiny, with warm highlights that serve as poignant reminders of lives foreshortened. We use cork collars to prop up skulls we are working on, so they will not roll and fall off the tables.

Skeletons in every phase of articulation are housed here, some lying full length on tables, some tucked away in fragments in boxes. A fetal skeleton, seven months developed and stillborn, stands in a bell jar, frail and pearly white, resembling a little monkey with its curiously bulbous skull, eggshell-thin, almost translucent. Jaws without teeth and teeth without jaws grin in ivory scatters. The dark, eyeless shadows of orbital sockets gaze calmly up at the ceiling or over at you. Bones creamy white, butterscotch yellow, dirty gray, sooty black, tangled and tumbled, boxed and loose, articulated and arrayed: a whole community of skeletons is kept here under lock and key, entrusted by chance and the state of Florida to my care.

This laboratory is my realm. It was built in 1991, by my design. I oversaw every detail: the 48-inch tube lights that can be clicked on and off in symmetrical pairs to vary room brightness; the twin, independent ventilation systems; the security locks which seal off the laboratory proper from the administrative area, every door, window and drain. The walls within the laboratory go all the way up to the roof, not just to the drop ceiling, for purposes of security as well as to isolate unpleasant odors.

Security is adamantine. There are burglar alarms strewn throughout the building, including motion detectors. The laboratory doors are fitted with Keso locks manufactured by the Sargent Lock Co. The keys do not have serrated edges, as normal keys have. Instead they are pocked with a unique pattern of depressions. The lock company will issue a duplicate key only upon receipt and verification of my signature. No one outside my staff possesses a key to the laboratory, not the college administration, not even the campus police. The laboratory is locked at night. Maintenance staff cannot enter it unless I am there.

Why this stern isolation? The contents of the laboratory, the bones and the equipment, are not so very valuable in terms of money. But some of them are legally irreplaceable: they represent potential evidence in court cases and must not be tampered with. A determined cracksman could doubtless cut his way in through the wall with the proper tools, but he would set off alarms and would leave a telltale hole, instantly communicating the fact that the precious bones were no longer inviolate, that the chain of evidence had been broken.

In one corner of the laboratory is a safety shower fitted with special nozzles. It sprays water in a powerful yet gentle stream, soft enough to point at your eye and wash it out, if you should happen to be hit with a spurt of formalin, acid or alcohol, all irritating chemicals familiar to those who deal with corpses in the laboratory.

Nearby are three "odor hoods," clear, ventilated enclosures, each large enough to accommodate a body on their stainless steel trays inside. The sinks came from photo supply stores and were meant to be used to develop pictures. Easy to flush clean, they are ideal for holding human remains that still have old flesh on them. The clear plastic hoods isolate odors and fans carry the corpse stench outdoors when the trays are occupied. Soft tissue removed from the bodies is placed in heat-sealed plastic bags and put in a freezer to one side. I and my students use sleeves of tubular plastic stock, supplied by the KAPAK Co. and made of 3M plastic. These can be cut and sealed to any length. Odors never penetrate the 4.5-mil thickness of the plastic. KAPAK heat-sealable pouches are used for smaller bits of flesh. These sturdy packets are, as their label proclaims, "FREEZABLE BOILABLE MICROWAVABLE AIRTIGHT." A portable impulse sealer looks like a paper cutter and is kept in a leather briefcase. Plug it in, lever down the arm and with a single stroke the plastic container is sealed hermetically.

There are times when you might walk into this room and know right away we've been working on something fresh. Sometimes the odors are ghastly. Sometimes, believe it or not, they are appetizing. Strange to say, when I was in my old laboratory in the Florida Museum of Natural History, people would come in and say: "What's cooking?" or "That sure smells good." When they found out it was a freshly burned human body they would go green and rush out.

———

" 'How long will a man lie i' the earth ere he rot?' " Prince Hamlet asks the gravedigger in the first scene of the fifth act of Shakespeare's great tragedy. " 'Faith,' " the gravedigger replies, " 'if he be not rotten before he die,—as we have many pocky corpses nowadays, that will scarce hold the laying—he will last you some eight year or nine year. . . .' "

Shakespeare was an unequaled observer of human nature, but decomposition depends on many variables. A buried corpse may last nearly forever in icy ground. Peat and moisture may also retard decay. In dry sand bodies will mummify to durable parchment. In mineral-rich earth they may be impregnated with salts and metals. But above the earth, especially in warm weather, the interval to skeletonization can be shockingly rapid. The minimum time of total skeletonization is not nine years, nor yet nine months, nor even nine weeks: it may occur in nine days or thereabouts. Dr. T. D. Stewart in his *Essentials of Forensic Anthropology* cites the case of a twelve-year-old girl who had been missing for ten days in Mississippi, following a hurricane. Her remains were found under a discarded, vinyl-covered sofa in the warm months of late summer, so the conditions for dissolution were almost optimal. It was as if she had been placed in a bug incubator. The bugs flourished, the remains diminished and in just over ten days the body had been very nearly skeletonized, with only a few small tabs of cartilage left.

In the late 1970s my colleague Bill Bass set up the Anthropological Research Facility (ARF) at the University of Tennessee at Knoxville. He began deliberately exposing bodies donated by the local medical examiner's office as unidentified or unclaimed to a carefully monitored process of natural corruption. It was a "decay rate facility," or, as my colleague Dr. Douglas Ubelaker calls it in his book, *Bones,* an "al fresco mortuary."

In this open-air morgue, thirty to forty bodies continue to be processed each year, along with a handful of dogs. The corpses are placed on concrete slabs or on the bare earth, or are wrapped in plastic or buried in shallow pits. Everything is photographed regularly, to monitor the process of dissolution. The buried bodies are exhumed at intervals, photographed, and reinterred. It's all for science, but local wags have added Bass's name to the acronym, renaming the facility "BARF."

Corpse reek is something you simply have to get used to in my profession. It is one thing to tell yourself that you are smelling butyric acid, methane gas and other organic compounds that are all quite common in nature. But it is quite another to see a clear and present horror lying upon the examining table, laughing with fleshless mouth, gazing with jellied eyes, a soul-flown shell, unstrung, inert, exanimate and ruined. I suppose there is a psychological element in the horror it excites in us, far beyond the actual, physical smell. It shouts "Death!" to our brains at some elemental level, and it takes experience and willpower to overcome the impulse to shrink away and flee. But I never put Mentholatum on my upper lip during an autopsy, the way the FBI agents did in the movie *Silence of the Lambs*. Nobody I know does. After a while you just think around it, think it away.

I have seen policemen, lawyers, x-ray technicians and others become ill and flee the room where such corpses lie, but I am proud to say not a single one of my students has ever flunked this stern trial of nerves. The only times I see my students bothered by such sights occur not in the grotesque, "Halloween" cases, where you see the decomposing skull with the remains of the eyes still glistening in place and tatters of flesh and cartilage adhering to bones; rather, it is the fresh bodies that tend to unsettle them.

Upon the table they see a homicide victim scarcely cold, who climbed from bed just as they did that day for the start of another busy day, who dressed and left her apartment, not knowing that in a few hours she was going to be murdered and would finish the day on the cold metal table in the pathologist's facility. These are the truly dreadful cases, in my students' eyes. There is the tendency for the student to look down and see not the victim, but themselves; to identify with the victim. And that can be one of the most emotionally wrenching experiences imaginable. It's easy not to identify with a skeleton or a grotesquely decomposing mass, or even a burned body, with its limbs contorted into the pose of a boxer as the roasted muscles have contracted amid the flames. Such miserable remains aren't "human" anymore. But the fresh body on the table can convey a terror beyond that of the most liquefied corpse.

There is no horrible, hidden mystery involved in decomposition. Basically there are two well-mapped processes involved: autolysis and putrefaction.

Autolysis occurs after death when digestive juices, which in life. dissolve only food, begin to digest the gastrointestinal tract. Within a few hours of death, these stomach acids will gnaw through the stomach or esophagus which they have patiently and obediently served through every moment of life. It is like some little French Revolution of the guts, in which the servants suddenly become the masters and run amok. At the same time tyrosine crystals may form in the liver as proteins there break down after death.

Putrefaction occurs as a result of bacterial activity throughout the body. Putrefaction is a much greater component of the decomposition process than autolysis, and it sweeps through the body like a silent fire. Blood is a fertile sea in which bacteria swarm and multiply. Gas is released within the blood vessels and tissues. The body swells, becomes distended with methane gas. The body can actually swell to two or three times its normal size in twelve to eighteen hours. A colleague of mine, who shall remain nameless, sometimes demonstrates this phenomenon for visitors by darkening his laboratory, lighting a match and thrusting a needle into the swollen set of remains. There is a great blue jet of flame and onlookers gasp.

As we dissolve, our skin color may change from green to purple to black. Dislodged by the pressure of the accumulating methane, our organs may bloom out from our lower orifices, and foul-smelling fluid may exude or spurt from these openings. The smell is largely composed of butyric acids—this is the stench of death that is so repellent to our nostrils. The skin slips from its moorings, so much that the skin of the hands can sometimes be removed completely, like a glove, though the nails fall away. Fingerprints can still be taken from these slipped-off "gloves." To do this, the technician must insert his own gloved hand into the dead bag of skin, ink the dead fingertips and carefully roll the prints onto a blank card.

It is a myth that fingernails and hair continue to grow after death. What really happens is that the skin may retract around them, making the hair and nails prickle up and jut out more prominently. Erich Maria Remarque, in his novel, *All Quiet on the Western Front*, imagines a dead friend's nails growing in weird, subterranean corkscrews after his burial. It is a powerful, disturbing image, but it is pure moonshine. No such thing occurs.

Dreadful as all these processes may seem, they are only the resolution of certain carbon-based compounds into certain other carbon-based compounds. Carbon is the element of life and death. We share it with diamonds and dandelions, with kerosene and kelp. While we may wrinkle our noses at some of its manifestations, we ought also to remember that this element comes to us from the stars, which wheel over us forever in silent, glittering array, pure fires obeying celestial laws.

Against another wall of my laboratory is my workbench, fitted with a drill press, a small anvil, saws, screwdrivers, wrenches and other tools. These implements are not for working with human remains, though their abstract shapes sometimes come in handy in unexpected ways. I use them to design frames and supports and other furniture for the laboratory. I am rather handy with tools, and it is satisfying to do this work myself.

My familiarity with tools often enables me to reach grim conclusions when I am working with the remains of murder and suicide victims. Sometimes I can tell exactly what sort of tool was used to kill someone. The cross section and the size will match up perfectly. I had a case recently in which a rubber mallet was used, just like the one on my toolbench wall. Another skull I examined was perforated with a pattern that perfectly matched the one on this pry bar. I often go to Sears and look at the tools there to see if any match up to the holes in the skulls that come to this laboratory. When the salesman asks: "Can I help you, sir?" I tell him, "No, you wouldn't understand. I'll know what I'm looking for when I see it."

Nearby you will see some machine grinders, used to grind down bones for samples; diamond-blade saws used to cut thin sections from bones and teeth so that they can be examined under a microscope; and the vibrating Stryker saw used in autopsies, a tool whose circular blade does not spin, but instead oscillates back and forth at high speed so that it will not cut skin, but only bone. The Stryker saw is used to cut the top of the skull off so that the brain can be removed. Garden tools such as branch cutters can be used to cut through ribs. Long knives are useful in removing the brain which, if fresh, leaves the skull reluctantly, with a sucking sound. But brain matter is quick to deliquesce and soon turns to a dark pudding.

A valuable array of photographic equipment is kept in the laboratory to take pictures of remains and bones. I only use High 8 Metal P videotape in my lab videocamera; it gives you videotapes of near studio quality. I also use a $5,000 Bronica camera with closeup accessories, similar to a Hasselblad but a bit cheaper, to take still pictures—*very* still pictures. The laboratory also has its own miniature x-ray machine, a Hewlett-Packard Faxitron 43805N and an x-ray duplicator, which can copy x-rays like a Xerox machine.

More than any other of my colleagues I use x-rays. Since we are not worried about harming the patient, we can leave the machine on for exposures of up to fifteen minutes, ending up with radiographs that shine through and through like gossamer membranes, not bone at all. There is no danger of overexposure. You cannot harm a dead skull with excessive x-rays, after all. That is our advantage. I prefer to use the same type of x-ray film that is used for mammography, as it is extremely sensitive and capable of showing extremely fine detail.

I'm always on the lookout for cheap equipment and I fancy I have rather a keen eye for a bargain: my twenty x-ray viewers were government surplus, bought from VA hospitals. They are so durable that I have not had to replace a single bulb in them yet. One particularly useful piece of equipment is a "hot spot" lamp, bought for ten dollars at a warehouse auction and capable of projecting a beam of light through the murkiest predeath x-ray films, illumining details that remain lost in shadows when exposed on an ordinary light table. These antemortem x-rays tend to be very dark and opaque because they are taken with extremely low levels of radiation, so as not to harm the living flesh. The "hot spot" pierces them, searches through their darkest shadows and blackest corners. It was the "hot spot" that enabled me to recognize a vital piece of evidence in my most vexing case, a crucial bit of rib from the Meek-Jennings murder-suicide case.

My students have to take a series of hepatitis B inoculations before they are permitted to work in the lab. We go through incredible numbers of disposable gloves, protective sleeves, shoe covers and smocks. Often, when working with especially ripe remains, two sets of gloves will be worn. Disposable plastic goggles are necessary when working with saws, and full plastic visors guard our faces against unexpected spurts and geysers of fluids too foul to describe, expelled by the pent-up gases of corruption. The laboratory has portable metal detectors, surveying equipment, shovels, rakes and archaeologists' trowels, to be used on field digs.

I greatly fear that anatomical expertise among medical doctors is on the decline, because of the crushing load of the modern medical curriculum and the shortage of skeletons. The former sources of skeletons, India and Bangladesh, have now prohibited their export, as an affront to national dignity. When I was a student myself, a first-class skeleton, with twenty-eight of thirty-two teeth still in place, with no damaged bones, articulated completely, mounted on a stand, with its muscle attachments painted in red and blue, all carefully labeled, would go for $600. Today such a skeleton, if you could find one for sale, would cost $3,000–5,000. Plastic reproductions are readily available, but the fine detail and texture are simply lacking from the plastic models. They are useless for all but the most rudimentary anatomical training. Current catalogs list plastic skeletons at $659.95. A first-class human skull, of real bone, not plastic, lists for $359. Whenever your self-esteem flags or fails, you can reflect that you are walking around with several thousand dollars' worth of bones encased within you, and that your skeleton is getting more valuable every year.

All of my students take what they call "the bone course," human osteology, in their junior or senior year. As they progress, I give them spot examinations. I begin by handing them ten large fragments of bone and allowing them a minute and a half to identify each one, to tell whether it is human, what bone it is, and whether or not it is the right or left bone. Then, as the semester progresses, the intervals of time get shorter and shorter, and the bits of bone get smaller and smaller. By the end of the term all ten samples can fit in a small matchbox.

Bones can riddle us devilishly. Often I try to fool my students by including fetal bones or bones from a bear's paw, which can look astonishingly human. I've been called out on two cases where "human hands" turned out to be bear paws. I have seen forensic pathologists identify lost bones in skulls as penetrating injuries by weapons. I've seen the bones of a blue heron gravely identified as human. I have seen specialists who should know better identify with great confidence the sex of a teenager incorrectly. I have seen sheep's ribs identified as human ribs. Turtle shells can cause terrible confusion, and gopher tortoises and snapping turtles are awful tricksters. Pieces of their shells look very like fragments of human skullcaps. Only recently I was called out to investigate some suspicious bone fragments found near a spot where a body had been found earlier. The police asked me if a serial killer were using this area as his dumping ground. I was able to reassure them immediately: the fresh "skull" was a crushed turtle shell.

It is one thing when we are fooled by nature's mimicry. It is quite another when a cunning skeletal hoax is put before the scientific community and passed off as a revolutionary discovery. Perhaps the most famous fraud ever attempted along these lines was the renowned skull of "Piltdown Man," which was "unearthed" early in

42

this century. I have held this extraordinary relic in my own two hands.

Piltdown Man was exposed as a manufactured pastiche in 1953. Even today it is remembered as a remarkable example of science gone awry, a bizarre plot excogitated by a pair of doctors for reasons that remain obscure. Harvard biologist Stephen Jay Gould has made a convincing case that the great Jesuit scientist and mystic, Teilhard de Chardin, very likely connived at the deception. Today we know nearly the full story: how the jaw of an ape, with its teeth carefully filed down, was joined to the skull fragments of a human; how it was buried secretly near a stately English mansion; how it was "unearthed" in 1911 near Piltdown and presented to the world as Piltdown Man, a unique specimen allegedly linking man with the apes.

Nowadays such a fraud would be spotted almost instantly. The filed-down teeth would stand out like a sore thumb under microscopic analysis, and fluorine tests would clearly show the skull and jaw were not of the same age. Fossils absorb fluorine from the earth at a steady rate and the wide discrepancy would have proved the jaw and skull fragments didn't match.

But in its heyday the skull of Piltdown Man was kept in a carefully guarded vault in the British Museum of Natural History as a national treasure, and only in the rarest circumstances was permission granted to study it. Most scholars had to content themselves with looking at a cast. Piltdown Man's skull was too precious to be touched or handled by the vulgar mob of ordinary researchers!

In 1966, when I was returning from Africa to begin my first teaching job in this country, I dropped in at the British Museum of Natural History to examine some baboon skulls there, some of which had been collected by L. S. B. Leakey in the 1920s. While I was at the museum I had a notion to ring up Dr. Kenneth Oakley, who had been instrumental in exposing the Piltdown Man hoax. Oakley very kindly invited me up to the collection area, where we had a friendly chat about Piltdown Man's skull and its strange history.

"Care to see it?" Oakley asked me offhandedly. How could I

pass up a chance to see this remarkable fake, which had exercised the ingenuity of some of the greatest anthropologists of all time? I agreed eagerly. To my utter amazement, Oakley turned, opened an ordinary filing cabinet, fished around in its depths and came up with the skull of Piltdown Man! As I handled the venerable, caramel-colored old fraud with its well-honed teeth, I could not help reflecting how low it had tumbled from its exalted rung on the ladder of evolution.

There are three women in particular who have had to deal with my extraordinary job more than any others: my wife Margaret and my two daughters, Lisa and Cynthia. I freely admit my job can make extraordinary demands on my marriage. Sometimes my wife made me take my clothes off and leave them on the washing machine before coming indoors. I can't argue with that. My daughters, especially Lisa, sometimes urged me to discuss my latest case over the dinner table, and my wife usually interposed a stern veto.

Once I convinced my wife to go with me in her car to pick up a decomposed body in Fort Myers. This was no small concession on her part, because this was her new car we'd be using, a Cadillac Cimarron. The body was very far gone and I disarticulated it at the office of the medical examiner, putting the portions into one very long bag, several feet long. Unfortunately one of the bones was broken and at some point when it was placed in the car, or soon afterward, the sharp bone punctured the bag and the contents leaked into the trunk. Bones can be very sharp. The bone in our Cadillac's trunk that day certainly was.

We began to notice an odor inside the car and found that it was better to drive with the windows down rather than using the air conditioning. By the time we got to Tampa the odor was very strong and we decided to stop for an early lunch at a Steak & Ale restaurant. We were fortunate to get a parking space near the front door and had our lunch. As we came from the restaurant and opened the front door, the odor from our car was extremely strong. I was surprised we hadn't been paged by the restaurant manager or that there were no police around.

We resumed our journey north. I happened to see vultures overhead. To this day I don't know if that was coincidental. Cadillac includes a rubber pad beneath the trunk liner, so it was possible to wash away most of the odor, but my wife could never look at that car again without remembering the episode. She traded in the car soon afterward, and she no longer allows me to use her car to pick up bodies.

Some gallows humor is inevitable when dealing with the dead, if only to deflect the sheer dread of what lies upon the examining table. I have seen this irreverent humor many times, but I do not permit it inside the C. A. Pound Human Identification Laboratory. I do not allow my students to dress up a skeleton, to put hats on skeletons, or to put cigarettes in their mouths. I do not allow them to give the skeletons humorous names, like Roscoe or Alphonse or anything of that nature.

Once when I was testifying in court a glib prosecutor tried to crack a joke about a mounted skeleton that had been introduced as a demonstrative model.

"What do you call this skeleton?" he asked me. "Do you have a pet name for him?"

"The skeleton," I answered. "I call him the skeleton." The courtroom spectators cracked up and the prosecutor was left very red-faced. But it is my belief that every set of remains deserves a certain minimum of respect. We owe them that.

"The Enfolding Earth"

Romeo: "Courage, man; the hurt cannot be much."

Mercutio: "No, 'tis not so deep as a well, nor so wide as a
church-door; but 'tis enough, 'twill serve: Ask for me tomorrow
and you shall find me a grave man. . . ."

—Shakespeare, *Romeo and Juliet,* Act III, Scene 1

A friend of mine, Dr. Michael Baden, the former chief medical examiner for New York City, is fond of saying that no burial is forever. Burial is only long-term storage. Newtonian physics teaches us that what goes up must come down, but where corpses are concerned, very often what goes down can come up again, and the sight can be passing strange. "Rest in Peace," we carve on our tombstones, heavy slabs of marble that are almost certainly destined to be scattered like chaff, long before the Last Judgment. When we consider that scarcely an active cemetery on the planet is more than a few hundred years old, we realize how short our undisturbed subterranean sleep can be.

"There is no antidote against the Opium of time," writes Sir Thomas Browne in his "Hydriotaphia." "Our Fathers finde their graves in our short memories, and sadly tell us how we may be buried in our Survivors. Grave-stones tell truth scarce fourty years: Generations passe while some trees stand, and old Families last not three Oaks. . . ."

I have assisted in many exhumations. I never cease to be amazed at the extraordinary things people do with dead bodies, the crazy, senseless methods they adopt to dispose of a corpse. In one of my cases a fellow buried his murdered girlfriend on the beach but left one of her legs sticking out of the sand so that she would be found and given a decent burial. In another, a murderer took three days to cremate a body in his backyard, tending the fire carefully until the cremation was as complete as it possibly could get—and then he turned himself in to the police. Perhaps he hoped to escape punishment by making the body unidentifiable. If so, he was sadly mistaken. I have a great deal of experience working with "cremains," and I identified it conclusively.

The burial container is terribly important. Sealed containers protecting the body from the environment, be they a sealed steel casket costing thousands of dollars or a cheap container made of plastic or Styrofoam, will result in an amazing degree of preservation, even over long periods of time. I've seen a well-embalmed body—an autopsied body, which makes embalming very difficult—last inside a sealed casket within a burial vault for twenty-seven years, looking as if death had taken place only a day or so before, with perfectly natural features and only small areas of skin slipping from the hands and feet. I have seen other bodies buried in wooden caskets that soon disintegrated, leaving the bones badly damaged, with virtually no remaining soft tissue. I had a case in which a newborn infant was wrapped in textiles, enclosed in a plastic bag, shut up in a vinyl suitcase and buried in sandy soil for ten years. When we excavated the remains we still found soft tissue preserved, keeping those tiny, delicate bones in their respective positions, preserving them as well as if they had belonged to a fresh body buried only a few weeks earlier.

Even unshielded by any container, a body will last longer underground. The general rule of thumb for the rate of decomposition is:

one week in the open air equals two weeks in water, equals eight weeks underground. The horrific picture of "worms" devouring a buried corpse is false. Flies will lay eggs on a body even before it is dead, and their wriggling, wormlike larvae, known as maggots, will hatch out in just under twenty-four hours. The cycle is so regular that it can sometimes be used to establish the time of death. But maggots cannot live underground. My colleague, Doug Ubelaker of the Smithsonian Institution, investigated an ancient Arikara Indian burial site in South Dakota and found that fly pupal cases were present in 16.4 percent to 38.3 percent of the burials at five sites, even though the burials were over two feet deep. How did they get there? Flies and beetles do not burrow more than a few inches below the ground. The answer is, the insects found their way to the corpse before it was buried, and were buried alive with it. When we examined the remains of Zachary Taylor, we found fly pupal cases among the bones. The industrious flies of Washington, D.C., had been at work on Taylor's body as it lay in state. They are no respecters of rank.

Maggots are tough, resourceful creatures. They have been known to feast on the remains of cyanide-poisoning victims and happily thrive on them. They have a covering of chitin that is almost impervious to everything but flamethrowers. They have evolved so as to live out their lives amid surroundings that would make most people faint with nausea; yet for them our corpses are delightful, a fragrant Elysium dripping with nectar and ambrosia. I have seen exultant maggots hopping like popcorn over the decaying remains of a human body, seething in glad myriads, leaping as high as eighteen inches in the air, falling on the floor with a soft, pattering noise, like gentle rainfall. They attack not at random but in concert, like shoals of hungry piranhas. I have known maggots to attack a body so zestfully that, over the space of a few hours, their combined jostling can shove the false teeth out of a dead man's mouth.

But let us leave our hungry little bugs and return underground. When all is said and done, burial is the most common means of disposing of a body, the method preferred by killers as well as innocent, ordinary citizens. A buried body can be devilishly difficult to find. In fact, except for the rare accident, buried bodies are seldom found, unless someone confesses to their whereabouts. Even then, it may prove extraordinarily difficult to locate the actual grave, because of changes in vegetation or terrain, or the confused state of mind of the individual who did the digging. "It was dark. I couldn't really see. I think it was around here somewhere"—these are the vague directions you most often hear. But if no one talks, and the burial remains secret, and the grave ages a bit, then finding a buried body is in truth the rarest of accidents. The killer who kills and buries the body without anyone's knowledge is safest from recovery of the remains. The more people present when the body was buried, the more likely it is to be found.

One of the strangest cases in my experience involved a body that had been buried by a multitude of people, nearly all of whom later helped us search for it, eagerly but without success. Over and over again those who witnessed the burial tried to lead police to the makeshift grave, in vain. It took a year to find the spot, even though police knew within a few weeks exactly who was in the grave and how he had come to be shot. He died, of all places, at a birthday party.

The victim had been an unfortunate young man, discharged from the military because of emotional problems. He had attacked his drill sergeant, and anyone who has served in the Army knows what a feckless deed that is. Some time after his discharge he attended a birthday party for a friend who was a parolee from a Florida prison. When the presents were unwrapped, one gift in particular caught the victim's eye: a holster for a .357 magnum revolver, given to the birthday boy by his girlfriend. The recipient proudly strapped on the holster and put the gun in it, wearing both while dancing at the party. For some reason, this gun and holster excited the keenest jealousy in the mind of the victim, who complained loudly that the guest of honor had such a beautiful gun, while he had none. Laughing, the birthday boy unbuckled the gun and holster, handed them to the victim and invited him to wear them. Greedily the victim snatched the revolver and holster, strapped them on and went outside. After a minute or two, the parolee followed him, perhaps because he was worried about losing his gun. A few seconds later a shot rang out.

Pale and distraught, the guest of honor rushed back into the house and announced that the victim had shot himself. The other guests rushed out and found the victim in a sitting position against the base of a tree, dead, dripping blood from a massive head injury, with the gun on the ground next to his limp hand.

Whether their wits were fogged by alcohol, or whether they were simply stupid I cannot tell; but instead of reporting the shooting to the police, the partygoers decided to place the body in a sleeping bag and transport it to the edge of the county, where they all helped bury it in the dark of night. It didn't take long for the story of the shooting to leak out—the parolee was charged with possession of a firearm by a convicted felon, failure to report a death and transporting a body from the scene of a death. He was sent back to prison and for a time it seemed he might be charged with murder.

The shooting occurred in late 1979, but the body was not unearthed until November 1980. It took the police over a year of tramping up and down in the woods before they found the grave. All this while, the penitent partygoers were racking their brains, trying to remember where they had mislaid the corpse. When it was finally unearthed, the skull of the victim was found to be reduced to approximately eighty fragments by the terrific explosive force of the .357 magnum slug, and it required extensive reconstruction at the C. A. Pound Human Identification Laboratory. Eventually I located the entrance wound and the well-defined and externally beveled exit wound. The trajectory of the bullet, which entered in the right temporal bone of the skull, was upward and slightly forward, consistent with the story of a self-inflicted gunshot wound.

If I had not been able to reconstruct that skull, very likely the birthday boy would have been charged with murder. As matters stood, he was sentenced to 186 days in jail and immediately released, with time served. He was relieved. At his sentencing he told the judge: "It's been riding me since 1979. I've had no comfort." To my knowledge, no other charges were ever filed against the partygoers, despite the macabre and unorthodox circumstances of their nocturnal trip to the woods.

In 1981 a sordid tale of brutality and child abuse was cut short by a well-aimed bullet from a .22-caliber rifle, leaving me with the buried body of a man in his forties, recovered from a shallow grave in central Florida. My analysis of the skull would help decide the fate of a seventeen-year-old girl who had confessed to shooting him.

The girl told police that she had been living in a hellish nightmare for eight years. She was the stepdaughter of the dead man and said he had been sexually abusing her since she was nine years old. She had an infant daughter, who was the child of this protracted, brutal union.

One night, the teenager told police, she was getting out of bed after being forced to submit to sex yet again, when her stepfather giggled oafishly: "I'm glad you had a daughter so I can break her in right." Something inside the girl snapped when she heard these words. She said she picked up a .22 rifle propped nearby, brought it up to her hip and shot her stepfather while he was standing a few feet away. Fearful she would be charged with murder, the girl persuaded her mother to help her tie up the wrists of the naked body, load it onto the back of their pickup truck, drive to a secluded spot and drag it about 185 yards into the woods, where they buried it.

A year passed. Finally the mother and daughter confessed to the crime and led police to the unmarked grave in the woods. We verified that the decomposed corpse was indeed that of the stepfather by a comparison of x-rays taken of him some years before his death with those taken of the recovered remains. I was asked to check the direction of the gunshot wound to see if it was consistent with the girl's story. I found a small-caliber gunshot wound perfectly centered between the eyes which then entered the braincase at a point that gave us the trajectory. It matched the girl's story with extraordinary exactitude. If he had been lying down, sitting down, standing to one side of her, or in any other position than the one she described, the bullet would almost certainly not have followed the path it did. She was telling the truth. We were able to determine that the bullet had traveled in a decidedly upward direction and that the victim had been directly facing the shooter.

I confess I had some difficulty dredging up any pity for the deceased in this case. The world lost little when he was murdered. Rather, my sympathies were entirely with the accused. It was a neat shot, to drill a man through the forehead with a rifle fired from the hip, and .22-caliber bullets are often too small to kill, even when fired at the head. The victim often ends up paralyzed, not dead. It was indeed a lucky piece of marksmanship.

After I submitted my findings to the authorities, the girl was charged as a youthful offender and placed in a juvenile facility, where she would receive counseling.

One of the most revolting, yet instructive, burial cases in my experience involved a terrible old man who lived in Miami and who finally died, aged ninety-five, a few years ago. This man was in the habit of threatening his neighbors with all sorts of dark menaces, telling anyone who would listen that he had murdered his son-in-law and disposed of the body in a septic tank, and he would do the same to anyone who crossed him.

No one took the old devil seriously, and he finally died. His house was sold, and the new owner opened the septic tank in the backyard, in order to clean it. The tank was a huge affair, ten feet long, with three concrete slabs over its inlet—and inside its dark, malodorous depths was found the half-skeletonized remains of a middle-aged man, with a .22-caliber bullet hole drilled neatly through the center of his forehead, right between the eyes. The old man had not been idly boasting: he really had murdered his son-in-law.

Septic tanks are common in Florida, where many neighborhoods still lack sewer lines. Few people have the stomach to look inside them, but they are interesting places, containing several widely disparate microenvironments. You would have to go to Hawaii to find the extraordinary range of atmospheric conditions that you encounter in a common septic tank, with its extremes of aridity and moisture, which in turn create conditions equally favorable to extraordinary preservation and extraordinary decay.

Within the average septic tank there is a large mass of dry material, which floats like a matted crust over the fluid below. The active decomposition takes place within the fluid, and on the underside of the mat. But above the mat all is quite dry, and beneath the fluid, at the very bottom of the tank, there is usually a very compact mass of clay and sand, devoid of oxygen. This dark world has its own peculiar fauna: very often, millions of cockroaches will scuttle and seethe in vast colonies above the mat, sometimes crawling up the drainpipes and back into the house above them.

The murdered son-in-law had been cast into the tank still clad in his shirt and trousers. There he had floated for years, face down, his hands and feet dangling down into the liquid. As the flesh on his limbs decomposed, the various bones gently fell away from the trunk and descended to the bottom of the tank, where they were embedded in the clay and sand, and in this oxygenless environment they were preserved from further decay. The skull, too, finally fell away as the neck vertebrae came loose and drifted down into the silt at the tank bottom.

But the rest of the body, which remained trapped in and above the mat for fifteen years, was badly damaged and almost unrecognizable. The cockroaches had nibbled at the upper surfaces, and the bacteria-rich fluid had gnawed away at the lower surfaces. They presented a scene of almost total dissolution.

But the preserved bones of the hands and feet, together with the skull, had survived and from these the unfortunate young man was finally and unequivocally identified. He had been missing for a decade and a half, and his homicidal father-in-law had been a spry old eighty years of age when he killed the younger man, single-handedly lifted the concrete slab at the entrance to the septic tank, and stuffed the body in. The aged murderer was beyond earthly justice, but the case of his missing son-in-law could finally be closed.

North Florida is rich in Indian burial mounds, and beautiful flint arrowheads and precious pottery centuries old can be found here in abundance. Unfortunately these ancient treasure troves are tempting targets for scavengers. My colleagues in the anthropology department at the Florida Museum of Natural History have no love for pot hunters, those destroyers of history who dig into archaeological sites in their unsystematic and destructive lust to recover Indian artifacts and historic relics for private collections. But one day in 1980 two pot hunters made a rare discovery indeed, one that aroused my interest: a recently buried body.

The pot hunters were digging in an area of Dixie County that had been previously combed through by hundreds of other amateur treasure seekers. It looked like a World War I battlefield, cratered and crisscrossed with trenches. This particular pair of pot hunters, not being very imaginative, were digging in a filled-in trench previously excavated by their predecessors—not exactly a promising place to find artifacts! Their search was rewarded anyway. They found a human corpse. Being the alert and astute observers that they were, they quickly realized that a buried Indian would not have a blond ponytail or be buried in a plastic garbage bag.

The pair hotfooted it back to their pickup truck and held a hasty conference on the tailgate. What should they do? Retrieve the body? Rebury the body? Go to the police? Say nothing? Have a beer? They opted for the beer.

Soothed and fortified by the foaming brew, they collected their thoughts. Then, suddenly, one pot hunter had a dreadful notion: what if the person who did this were watching them right that minute from the woods? Flinging down their beer cans in panic, they beat a hasty retreat to the sheriff's office. Better confess to illegal pot hunting than connive at concealing a murder!

The sheriff's office called the Florida Department of Law Enforcement and the FDLE called me, asking that I cooperate in the excavation of remains. A curious scene ensued. The pot hunters were allowed by the sheriff to watch us while we excavated the mound, and they frequently pointed out bits of Indian chert or flint that I had uncovered. Watching me carefully work with my Marshalltown trowel, the trowel of choice for most professional archaeologists, one turned to the other and said: "Look! They use the same tools we do!"

At last came the grim task of examining the remains. The body was that of a female and the plastic garbage bag had preserved her soft tissues. Facial recognition even of a fresh body is difficult because of postmortem changes. That's the reason garbage bags are so helpful to us. They enclose the remains in a sealed, watertight environment, so the soft tissues last longer. The tissues are not beautiful, nor do they delight the nose, but they are recognizable.

We got a good description from the remains of the deceased and good evidence of the injuries she received at the time of her death. Even so, we had some difficulty learning her name. The body was still clad in a T-shirt with the words "PIGGLY WIGGLY" stenciled on it. Piggly Wiggly stores are popular supermarkets in many parts of the South. Now, the only Piggly Wiggly store within a hundred miles of the old Indian mound was in a nearby town. Police visited the store, spoke with the manager, asked when the shirt was sold, how many were sold. They did not think to ask if any employee had worn such a shirt, or if any of the staff was missing. Then they gave up.

So a specialist in artistic reconstruction of the face was called in. She came to my laboratory and got the information she needed. Facial reconstructions are not a new technique; people have been attempting to do them since the very early years of the nineteenth century. Today they are still a hotly debated procedure, nearly always a last resort. Some forensic anthropologists do them, some don't. As a rule, I don't. But in rare cases, when all other avenues have been explored without success, and when there are absolutely no more names of possible victims to investigate, then a reconstruction of the deceased's face can be of some value. If it is published in the newspaper, people may come forward and suggest one or more names of people they knew, who might have resembled the published image. A dead-ended investigation can thus be strung out a bit further, with a few more names to investigate, a few more persons to check out, a few more sets of records to compare to the remains. Sometimes it works. This was one of those times.

The reconstruction was published in a newspaper complete with a description that I provided and the fact that she was wearing a Piggly Wiggly T-shirt. The grandmother of a young woman phoned and reported that the image looked like her granddaughter. She was right. The body was, in fact, that of her granddaughter, who had worked at that Piggly Wiggly when she disappeared. We were able to match the granddaughter's dental x-rays with those of the remains.

Unfortunately no one was ever brought to justice for this murder. There was a very likely suspect, but there never was enough evidence for an arrest. At one level the case was solved. At another, it will never be solved. We have had no choice but to release the skeletal remains for burial, since it appears no trial will ever be held.

The macabre case of the La Belle drug murders was one of the most chilling ever to come to my attention. It occurred in 1981 and was one of the first illicit burials I investigated, but the grim details of the killings, which emerged little by little as the corpses were excavated over the course of a week, comprised a steadily unfolding tableau of horror.

My involvement began when I received a phone call from Dr. Wally Graves, the district medical examiner in Fort Myers. Wally told me the police had located the gravesite of three buried bodies. A team from the FDLE had already been assisting in the investigation. He told me that this was a drug case, in which three Northeastern businessmen had come down to Florida to negotiate with some local drug smugglers. As often happens in these sordid cases, negotiations broke down. The three Northeasterners were kidnapped from their hotel in Fort Myers and eventually shot and buried. All this had been learned from an informant who had turned state's evidence. The corpses would have to be disinterred very carefully if a case were to be made against their murderers. The details of the crime would have to be reconstructed from the stratigraphic evidence of the scene. The three individuals had been placed in a hole one at a time, shot, and then buried. The three corpses had lain in the grave pit for three years, one atop the other, like the levels of an ancient city. The whole excavation process turned out to be amazingly complex. Moreover, it had to be carried out in strictest secrecy. Everybody concerned fervently hoped that word of our activities wouldn't leak out, not only for the sake of the informant's safety, but for our own as well.

I had the happy thought of suggesting that I bring along a professional archaeologist to supervise the excavation. Wally and the FDLE agreed, and Dr. Brenda Sigler-Eisenberg of the Florida Museum of Natural History accompanied me.

Every morning I would check our car for disturbances of the hood and check beneath it for any sign of tampering. It did not escape me that we were staying at the same hotel from which the three drug dealers had been kidnapped.

To get to the site we had to drive through a golf course. When we arrived we found the local sheriff on hand, along with a number of investigators from the state attorney's office, several of whom guarded the dig site around the clock, armed with assault rifles. Investigators from FDLE and the FDLE crime scene analysts were also present and we soon settled into a workmanlike routine of digging and photographing and diagraming the hole and its grisly contents. We had the local fire chief there with a pumper truck to provide a water source to wash the gummy soil through screens so that we could recover all evidence, no matter how small.

The skull of the first body had been located before we got there. A shovel had shaved along the very top surface of the dry bone and we could see about a three-inch circular patch of exposed cranium. We began the excavation downward from there after establishing our grid system and our depth controls. The district medical examiner and one of his senior staff members pitched in, carrying buckets of dirt, washing the material through the screens, wearing oversized rubber boots. At first there was a rigid division of labor, but pretty soon everybody pitched in and we made good progress.

As the pit was slowly excavated over the next few days we began to see grim things. The uppermost body was that of a man whose hands were tied tightly behind his back. His body was arched like a bow since the other end of the rope was tied to his ankles. The head was encircled with duct tape around the mouth and showed clear evidence of a shotgun wound, from a gun fired at close range. Some skin remained on some of the lower parts of the body. It was eerie to watch as the color of the skin visibly changed to a darkening red as it was exposed to the sun and air, as if the long-decayed flesh were returning to a mocking semblance of life.

The body beneath him was face down. A rope was tied to one hand but did not secure the other limbs. He too had duct tape around his mouth. He had been shot in the upper right chest, from the front, and then had fallen downward over the third body. His arm was flung over the third body, which lay lowest in the grave.

In those days I was having some back trouble. I found it excruciating to stoop over these corpses for hours on end. I compromised by crawling down into the hole and lying alongside the bodies, digging them out while lying next to them, face to face. My unorthodox methods amused many of the investigators, as well as the medical examiner, who delighted in photographing me, lying alongside corpses, holding a trowel in one hand and a can of Dr Pepper soda in the other.

We found that our clothes were quickly becoming soiled and malodorous from working in the grave. We had to buy new clothes and have the hotel launder the ones we had been wearing. The hotel staff were extremely reluctant to handle our clothes at first, but after we explained to them the need they were very understanding. So we were able to wear fresh, clean clothes every day.

As time stretched on the investigators grew increasingly restless. At one point Dr. Sigler-Eisenberg announced that we needed some teaspoons so that we could clean away the soil around the bodies even more carefully. I thought we were going to have a full-scale revolt on our hands!

Dr. Sigler-Eisenberg's zeal impressed us all. She insisted on working straight through and not stopping for lunch even though we had sandwiches brought out to the site each day. Only later did I discover that she was too nauseated to eat.

While we were digging one day we heard that word of our activities had leaked out to the drug lords in Miami. Three carloads of them were said to be heading our way. I wondered what we would do if three carloads of men armed with automatic weapons drove onto the site. My first inclination would have been to jump into the hole with the three bodies, but then I realized that the most logical thing for the killers to do would be to throw explosives into the grave to destroy the evidence. Fortunately I never did have to decide what the best course of action might be. I suppose it would have been to run into the nearby palmettos to join the rattlesnakes.

The third body, which lay beneath the other two, was fairly well preserved. His organs could be discerned at the subsequent autopsy. As a rule, the deeper a body lies in the earth, the better the preservation. During the excavation we found small plastic wrappers that had encircled buckshot in shotgun shells. By the location of these wrappers, on top of the bodies and between them, we were able to establish the sequence of events.

The body buried deepest had been shot *last,* not first. Our conclusion was later corroborated by the informant, who later testified in court that the man who lay bottommost in the grave was actually the last to die. After the men were kidnapped from their hotel, they realized their situation was hopeless, that they were all going to die. Contemplating his fate, knowing that there was no escape, the third man had begged to be executed first, so that he would not have to watch the other two murders. In an exquisite refinement of cruelty, his tormentors threw him into the hole face up first, alive, shot his two colleagues so they would fall on him, and only then did they shoot him through the V of his open-necked shirt. He was the first to be buried, but the last to expire. His state of mind, as he was flung into the pit alive, as he heard the shots ring out, as he felt the bodies of his comrades fall on him, twitching and bleeding, I leave to your conjecture.

As a result of our excavation, whose results were reinforced by the informant's testimony in court, close to twenty people went to jail for various offenses related to drug trafficking and murder. I was relieved to see them there. The actual trigger man was a thug named Larry Ferguson (though the use of the word "thug" to describe this case is an insult to the memory of the bold, strangling assassins who practiced *thuggee* in India in the early nineteenth century). Ferguson went to trial, was found guilty of second-degree murder and received a prison sentence of twenty-one years.

All this lay in the future. When we finished our work in the murder pit and the bodies were taken away, one of the investigators from the state attorney's office shot a wild hog. We barbecued it near the excavation and feasted that evening on a somewhat tough but tasty barbecued pig, with baked beans and swamp cabbage. Dr. Sigler-Eisenberg seemed to regain her appetite at last.

Flotsam and Jetsam

TIN WOODMAN: "What happened to you?"

SCARECROW: "They tore my legs off and they threw them over there! Then they took my chest out and they threw it over there!"

TIN WOODMAN: "Well, that's you all over."

COWARDLY LION: "They sure knocked the stuffings out of you, didn't they?"

SCARECROW: "Don't stand there talking! Put me together!"

—The Wizard of Oz, 1939 MGM screenplay by Noel Langley, Florence Ryerson and Edgar Allan Woolf

To profane a dead body by cutting it to pieces has always seemed, at least to our Western eyes, an act of bestial brutality. It is one thing to do murder. It is quite another to destroy the murder victim's identity, and this is the effect of dismemberment. The Roman poet Vergil moves us to pity with his description of the death and decapitation of King Priam, after the fall of Troy, in the second book of the *Aeneid.* The king has lost his life but, what is worse, he has lost his selfhood.

Flotsam and Jetsam

*He, who was once lord of so many tribes and lands, the
monarch of Asia—he lies a huge trunk upon the shore, his head
severed from his shoulders, a corpse without a name!*

I see about four or five dismemberment cases a year, and they
are among the most challenging and frustrating crimes in my experience. I am not counting the accidental cases, which are caused by
car crashes or other mishaps involving machinery. I mean murder
victims who have been coldly, deliberately cut to pieces, whose frag-
mented bodies show the work of human malevolence—and hard
work at that. Taking apart a fresh human body is no mean task. You
will work up a sweat doing it. I have seen every tool imaginable used
for this grisly purpose, from the ancient stone choppers used by
early man millions of years ago in the Olduvai Gorge in Kenya to the
Rambo knives, hacksaws and chain saws of today. It is a bloody,
messy, dangerous business. Saws and knives can slip and wound you
while you are using them. Bone itself can be quite sharp; I have
been cut by broken bones while working with remains. The disease
of AIDS has made us all far more careful in the autopsy room; and
AIDS has created a new wrinkle in dismemberment cases. If the saw
blade were to slip and cut a murderer while he was cutting up a
victim afflicted with AIDS, he could quite possibly catch the disease.
In this case, the victim would be revenged on his killer, even after
death!

Alas, it must be admitted from the outset that dismemberment is
an extremely effective means of concealing a victim's identity. In this
chapter, I warn the reader fairly and beforehand, the riddles will
outnumber the solutions, and the scattered remnants of many of
these victims must await the Last Judgment, to be reunited and
speak the truth about their final hours.

Dismemberment cases are often lit with a baleful, lurid light in
my mind. In most of my cases I have to place myself in the role of
the victim, to see what happened at the time of death. I imagine the
gun firing at me, or the knife, or the hammer, or the ax, rising and

falling, sinking into my body. The victim and I, we are trying to defend ourselves. We throw our forearms up, we grapple with our fingers, we turn our heads aside, clinging to life. In such cases I relive the crime from the victim's standpoint, and the victim is very personified and individualized.

But in dismemberment cases the victim is already dead, and I must place myself inside the brain of the murderer, who has slain his victim and who is now cutting him to pieces. I become the dismemberer, imagining the scene, the tools, the strokes that hack the body asunder. "Why did you cut there?" I ask myself. "What implement did you use to do this? Did you pause to catch your breath? Were you in a hurry? Did you fling down one tool in disgust and seize another?"

Many dismemberments are done in bathtubs—more things come out of bathtubs than bathtub gin, I assure you!—and most of my cases seem to involve motorcycle gang members or people involved in the drug trade. The cases seem to cluster along the I-95 corridor in Florida, and if the state has a Dismemberment Capital, it is probably Daytona Beach. Interstate highways are the veins and arteries by which crime circulates in America. Serial killers seem to float through them like blood cells, sometimes fast, sometimes slow. Crimes committed along interstate highways ought to be considered extraterritorially, apart from the normal rules of geography, and separate from a state's good name. These huge highways form a kind of fifty-first state of their own, a state whose flower is the deadly nightshade and whose state bird is the vulture.

When I first got into forensic anthropology people tended to use hacksaws to dismember bodies. They were the tool of choice for killers because they are easily available, easily disposable, and their fine, serrated blades cut very efficiently through bone. It is a lot easier to saw through a human bone with a hacksaw than with a wood saw. I have verified this myself.

On the other hand, hacksaws are a great help to us who investigate such dismemberments. Very often a new hacksaw blade will leave a smear of paint on the bone surfaces—gray, orange, blue, yellow. Such smears can be analyzed chemically and very often matched up to a specific brand of saw blade.

In recent years, however, hacksaws have been supplanted by chain saws. Chain saws have certain advantages: the killer saves time and effort with a chain saw. But of course the disadvantage is that chain saws are incredibly loud and messy. They sling sprays of blood and debris in all directions. Chain saws, too, yield evidence to the eye of the experienced investigator. Often their cuts are quite individualized, differing noticeably from one model to the next. Sometimes we can even recover chain-saw oil from the bone surfaces which can be chemically analyzed. Although I have not heard of it done yet, there will undoubtedly come a day when the debris left over by a chain saw after a dismemberment, or even minute traces of flesh, bone and blood on the chain-saw blade itself, will be analyzed for their DNA content and matched up with the DNA of the victim.

In the collection of the C. A. Pound Human Identification Laboratory is a special set of cow bones which is very precious to me. As my experience with dismemberments increased, I decided it would be useful to have a catalog of saw marks as a sort of reference library. I therefore asked a technician at the Florida Museum of Natural History to do me a favor. I took him a box of fresh soup bones and asked him to saw through them with every type of saw we could think of: kitchen saws, table saws, wood saws, band saws, hacksaws, crosscut saws, pruning saws, chain saws, even anatomical Stryker saws, whose oscillating blade is designed to cut through bone, but not flesh. Under microscopic analysis every different type of saw will make a different type of tooth pattern in bone. A Stryker saw, for example, produces circular arcs of short radius, with some overlapping. A band saw's cut is very smooth. It leaves few tooth marks and those it does leave tend to be straight, fine and seldom overlapping. Hacksaw blade marks often overlap, because the person doing the sawing will change the angle of attack as he cuts through the bone. They look like a tiny, skewed tic-tac-toe board with thousands of squares. Chain-saw marks go straight through bone. A table saw with a rotating eight-inch blade, the kind a handyman might have mounted on his worktable, produces parallel curves. We labeled and photographed all these cut-patterns carefully. The collection is a valuable resource, though by now I carry most of the patterns in my head.

Anyone who has carved a chicken or a turkey knows that it is much easier to cut through the joint than through the solid bone. But you would be amazed how few dismemberers actually remove the legs at the hip. Most of them saw through at crotch level, leaving a stump of thighbone still attached to the pelvis, usually several inches long. This stump is a godsend to the investigator. It is here that we look for our saw marks. This upper leg bone, the femur, has very thick walls at this point and these walls often furnish very clear evidence of the implement used to cut through them. Thin-walled bones aren't nearly as good for this purpose. Even if a knife is used to disarticulate the joints, it will leave telltale gashes as well. My point is, there is no way to cut a body up and leave no traces of the tools you use. Hew at them though you may, bones yet will have their say.

In 1981, I was called to a medical examiner's office in Leesburg, in central Florida's Lake County. There I heard an extraordinary tale. It seems someone had observed a furry white dog, of a poodle-like breed, eating something on the side of the road. It developed that the dog was nibbling on the lower portion of a left human leg, very fresh. The dog had been hungry, and most of the muscle tissue was already devoured. A week later the lower portion of a right leg was found near Daytona, in Volusia County, over a hundred miles away.

When I compared these legs I found that they were very consistent with one another and almost certainly came from the same body. One of the most telling signs appeared on the knees: the skin below the knees showed a matching pair of calluses, of the type commonly seen on the knees of surfers. The legs had been chopped off an inch or so above the knee joint, the cuts passing through the lower kneebones at the same height on both legs. Microscopic analysis of the cut bone surfaces showed the fine straight marks of teeth that overlapped one another, as if the angle of attack had changed during manual sawing. This was a classic hacksaw dismemberment.

Alas, the surfer's legs were all of him that ever turned up. We never did find any other portion of that body, nor were we ever able to match a name to the remains. The route of the car could be ascertained fairly easily from the pattern of highways between the two far-flung legs. I made sure every sheriff's office along the way was notified of the case and asked them to be on the lookout for more remains. But none was ever found.

Many of these slayings were drug-related, and organized crime has more murder experience than any other segment of society. They know how to kill, and they know how to cover their tracks.

So it was in the case of the torso with the Grim Reaper tattoo. In 1987, I was invited to examine a headless, armless, legless trunk, upon whose shoulder was tattooed a large, detailed and horrific picture of the Grim Reaper, wielding his scythe, his bony jaws open in laughter. Neither the head nor the limbs were ever found, but we had high hopes that the tattoo would identify the torso. Tattoos are visible for long periods after death, almost as long as any skin remains on the body. Indeed, when the outer layer of skin, the epidermis, slips off in early decomposition, the underlying layers of skin, where the tattoo ink actually is, are exposed, making the colors much brighter and more vivid than during life. Many medical examiners actually keep photo libraries of tattoos taken from dead bodies to aid them in identifying remains, and this tattoo certainly belonged in a museum. It stood forth in blazing Technicolor. It was wonderfully distinctive. The police showed photographs of it around at all the bars frequented by bikers and their hangers-on. But no one remembered seeing it—or at least no one would admit to having seen it. The body was never identified. The Grim Reaper mocked us all with his fleshless jaws.

Left unattended, our defunct bodies quickly become part of the food chain. On land, flies, beetles, cockroaches, rats, dogs, cats, pigs, raccoons, bears and any number of animals rush in and feast whenever death rings the dinner gong. In water, alligators, fish, crabs and sharks are no less hungry. In such cases, the investigator practically has to elbow his way through a crowd of famished banqueters before he can salvage and examine what is left.

One case that gave me some difficulty was a body found in two pieces, washed ashore in different locations in the Florida Keys. The head and portions of the neck were found in one spot and nearly all the rest—the torso, with legs attached and feet cut partly away—in another. It appeared that sharks had bitten at, but not quite through, the neck. There were clear marks of sharks' teeth on the remains. But there were also very fine marks on the neck vertebrae still visible, which showed that the head had been sawed off. When I looked at the top vertebra protruding from the torso I saw similar marks which left no doubt: the body had been dismembered before it was thrown into the water. We were dealing with a murder, perhaps committed aboard a ship, and not a shark attack in the open sea.

I concluded that in this case a saw, probably a hacksaw, was used to dismember the body into three pieces, only two of which were ever found. Since both these fragments showed shark damage, I believe a shark got the rest of the corpse. Neither the victim nor his murderer was ever identified in this case, but at least we knew the killer was another human being, not a shark.

The shark, incidentally, is one of the true scavengers of the sea, and from time to time portions of human remains are found in sharks' bellies, but only if the shark is caught and cut open soon after swallowing them. The stomach acid of the shark's digestive system is extremely corrosive. It dissolves bone so quickly that the window of opportunity to find remains inside a shark is very small. A tibia I once examined, which had been taken from a shark's stomach, was reduced to a paper-thin cylinder of bone, with a greatly reduced diameter. It was so eaten away that investigators originally believed it was an ulna, a bone from the arm. I was able to set them straight: it was a tibia, a leg bone, dissolved to a shadow of itself by acid. Of all sharks, tiger sharks are fondest of human flesh. They are the species whose entrails most often yield up human remains.

In March 1990, I was called back in on a case involving a severed head that had been found in October 1987, in a closed vinyl bucket on the east coast of Florida, in Palm Beach County. For three years the head had been kept at the Palm Beach County medical examiner's office, awaiting identification or a lucky break in the case. The medical examiner's patience was finally rewarded. He learned that in 1983, four years before the head came to light, a headless trunk had been found clear across the Florida peninsula, propped against a pasture fence in a field belonging to a former county sheriff. A chain saw had been used to cut the head from the body.

Even though the two pieces were separated by many miles and several years, this case nevertheless resulted in one of the neatest match-ups of any dismemberment in my experience. The head had been cut off just below the hyoid bone, or Adam's apple. The neck ended just above the thyroid cartilage. By superimposing old x-rays, taken of the torso four years earlier, and new ones taken of the head (which had been very well preserved in its sealed vinyl bucket), we were able to prove they belonged together. The victim was identified as a Jamaican who had reportedly been involved in drug smuggling. In this case we were able to come up with a name for the victim and to take the head and body off the police's books. But his murderer escaped unpunished. No one was ever charged with this death.

The following month I received a complete body in two portions in the small and large suitcases of a set of matching luggage bought at Sears. The suitcases in this case were of the Hercules brand and were found in two different counties, miles apart: West Palm Beach in Palm Beach County and Fort Pierce in Martin County.

The body was cut in two through the lower back, at the top of the fifth lumbar vertebra. This was a somewhat unusual but not entirely unknown method of dismemberment. It all depends how many portions you want. If you are going to be frugal and make only one cut, the lower back is obviously the place you would choose.

In this particular case, however, the lower portion of the body had been further dismembered through the thighs. The dismemberment was probably done with a fine-toothed saw, such as a hacksaw. The torso of the upper portion of the body was wearing a T-shirt advertising the Boot Hill Saloon, a bar in Daytona popular with motorcycle enthusiasts. The victim was identified as a biker, but again no one was ever charged with his murder. Obviously he was the victim of gang justice, and his killers scattered his remains after cutting him to pieces and packing him up into the twin suitcases for his final trip.

By now the reader will perhaps share some of my frustration over these dismemberment cases. Over and over again I have acted the part of "all the king's horses and all the king's men" in the old Mother Goose rhyme, trying to reassemble some poor Humpty-Dumpty of a murder victim, who didn't fall off a wall, but who was most likely shot or stabbed to death, then laboriously sawed to pieces by his killer. At great pains, and against long odds, I have sometimes succeeded in reuniting pieces of bodies that seemed impossibly far-flung. Sometimes I can even make out the personality of the murderer and the circumstances of the crime. I can see a mental picture of the corpse cutter at work, panting and sweating, his teeth gritted, removing the head and limbs, one after another, with tools I can clearly identify. But all this is not enough. The pieces remain, the culprit goes uncaptured and unpunished.

The real victory in these dismemberment cases is often scientific and intellectual, rather than moral. More and more today, dismemberment cases are being treated with the attention they deserve. Under the old coroner system, nobody would look twice at a dismemberment. They were too puzzling and horrible to contemplate for long. A finding of "Body Taken Apart" would be entered, the remains would be buried and that would be the end of it. Now we are studying these appalling cases more and more closely, with a clearer knowledge of anatomy and with improved scientific techniques. As I have shown, we are sometimes able to piece together bodies that have been scattered practically to the four winds, across hundreds of miles; bodies lost for many years. It is not every day that we have the satisfaction of seeing a murderer and corpse cutter convicted and led away in handcuffs as a result of our work, but we are making progress.

One of the ghastliest cases of dismemberment I ever encountered ended in the most satisfying way imaginable, with a dramatic plea of guilty within minutes of my testimony. I call it "The Case of the Pale-Faced Indian." It happened this way:

In 1981, right after I'd finished helping dig up the bodies of the three drug smugglers down in La Belle, I was called in to identify a buried, dismembered body. The body belonged to a Gainesville man who owned land in a rural area. On this lot stood an unused house trailer. A Vietnam veteran named Tim Burgess, a desperate-looking man with long dark hair and flowing muttonchop whiskers, had asked permission to camp on the man's property. The landowner agreed, but Burgess soon took advantage of his hospitality and moved into the vacant trailer. When the landowner finally asked him to leave, Burgess refused.

The landowner learned that Burgess had a criminal record and had been paroled from prison. He had been arrested several times. Once, while walking a pet Doberman in front of the White House in Washington, D.C., his dog had lunged at a passerby and Burgess's coat had flapped open, revealing .45-caliber automatics and several hundred rounds of ammunition.

In short, Burgess was a creepy customer, a man with a violent past whose very sanity was open to question. Not wanting to confront him face to face, his reluctant landlord wrote a letter to Burgess's probation officer. He complained that not only was Burgess squatting on his property without permission but he was also growing marijuana in the woods.

I have long since ceased to be amazed at the extraordinary quirks of our criminal justice system. The probation officer, a soft-hearted sort, did nothing more than write Burgess a letter revealing that his landlord had complained about him. In the same letter was a stern warning to Burgess—to destroy his marijuana crop.

This letter was the unfortunate landowner's death warrant.

Completely unaware that Burgess was furious with him for tat-tling to his probation officer, the exasperated landowner went out to confront his trespassing tenant and have it out with him once and for all. He took his pet dog with him. Neither he nor the dog was ever seen alive again. When the landowner was reported missing a few days later, deputies went out to the property. There they found the victim's pickup truck and his dead dog. As they searched the prop-erty, an investigator tripped over what appeared to be a stick pro-truding up at an odd angle from the ground. Closer inspection re-vealed it was no stick but the severed end of a human thighbone, with the flesh rotted, dried and retracted from it.

(An odd sidelight: a few months later, when the same investiga-tor stepped into another patch of woods to relieve his bladder, he happened to discover *another* body. He had been searching for it for months, in a completely unrelated case. You would be amazed how many bodies turn up during these errands of nature; the body of the baby son of the famous aviator, Charles Lindbergh, was found by a truck driver in similar circumstances after the child was kidnapped in 1932.)

But to return to the bone protruding from the dirt: together with my archaeologist colleague, Dr. Sigler-Eisenberg, we set about dig-ging up the remains. Both thighbones had been cut through and the legs placed alongside the torso in the grave. There was one rather shocking detail: the victim had been scalped, with the hair and soft tissue cut away from the entire top of the head. The body also showed evidence of shotgun wounds to the buttocks, the abdomen and the neck. He had been killed with three separate blasts.

Burgess had fled, but not far. He was reportedly seen going into the woods with a .357 magnum revolver a mile away from the spot where we were excavating. Immediately all the investigators rushed pell-mell from the scene, eager to catch the prime suspect. As the last of them faded from view, Dr. Sigler-Eisenberg and I looked at each other. We both realized that we were defenseless, alone at the scene of a terrible murder, with the probable murderer roaming in the woods nearby! We waited in some suspense until the officers returned a short time later—only to make themselves scarce again when it came time to hoist the rotting remnants into our vehicle. It is amazing how burly policemen can dwindle and disappear when there is dirty work like this to be done!

Burgess's capture was a bit anticlimactic. While the search was still under way, he telephoned a neighbor who was a deputy sheriff and arranged to surrender to him personally.

The method of dismemberment in this case was unorthodox. Marks on one femur indicated that a knife was used to cut through the skin and muscle; then the knife was used to hack on the bones. If you have ever tried to use a large pocket knife or hunting knife to hack through a tree limb, you'll find that at first it appears you are making great progress, but after a while your arm is tired and you are still no more than halfway through. The same thing seems to have happened here. Weary and frustrated, the killer then went for an ax and finished the amputation with a single ax blow. Having served his apprenticeship on one leg, he then proceeded with the ax to the second leg, which he also severed.

But the grotesque multiple methods used to chop up the corpse paled in comparison with the grotesque theories Burgess's defense attorney raised at the trial. I have never seen a trapped man wriggle more artfully in court than Burgess did, through his lawyer. He pleaded not guilty to the charge of murder. He claimed he had acted in self-defense.

Burgess, his lawyer explained, believed he was an American Indian. The fact that he had scalped his victim proved that he had killed his opponent in self-defense, for Indians do not scalp helpless, unarmed people but only those whom they have slain in battle after a fair fight! I have never heard a more astonishing and original defense. The prosecutor actually arranged to call an ethnologist to the witness stand, to testify that this was absurd, that Indians had often taken scalps indiscriminately, even from victims they had not themselves killed, even from victims who remained alive after the scalping.

Then came my turn to testify. More than most others, dismemberment cases are an ordeal to testify about in court. I have to reveal in excruciating and grisly detail what exactly it is that I have learned from a set of human remains. As I speak, the court is hearing terrible things. The judge hears, the jury hears, the defendant hears—and oftentimes the mother, or father, or some other near, dear relative of the victim is listening to my testimony too, listening with tears trickling down their cheeks. At such times I cannot bear to think about the families. I shut them out from my mind. I focus on the remains, only the remains. They, not the living, are my sole concern. When a conviction does occur, it comes too late for the victim and is often scant comfort to the bereaved families. But it does help the future, potential victims of the killer, whose lives would be forfeit if he were not caught and punished.

But this time the dreadful recital of details had an astonishing result. I demonstrated to the jury with a folding hunting knife found in Burgess's possession exactly how he would have had to hold the very end of the handle to get sufficient leverage to hack at the bones and cause the damage I had observed. My testimony was sharply challenged by the defense, so I had to go over it again and again, with much repetition, and explanations, and repeated demonstrations.

All this while, Burgess was fidgeting in his chair. After I finished my testimony, and the medical examiner was beginning his, the accused motioned to his attorney. A whispered conference ensued. At the end of it, Burgess's attorney asked to approach the bench.

Burgess wished to change his plea to "guilty." His attorney explained that Burgess found the demonstrations of the death and dismemberment of his former landlord so true to life, so evocative of the real event, that it was recalling memories too horrible for him to bear.

Hearing this, I confess I felt a thrill of vindication. It's always damnably frustrating, at a trial, to know that the person in the court-room most able to confirm your testimony about a crime, the person who knows every single detail about it, is very likely the person on trial. He is sitting a few feet away from you, often staring right at you —but his lips are sealed forever. This case made up for many of the puzzling dismemberments which ended, after so much work on my part, in perplexity and riddles. This time at least, like the heavy clang and click of a prison door slamming shut, there was the satisfying sense of absolute certainty.

6

"When the Sickness Is Your Soul"

If it chance your eye offend you,
Pluck it out, lad, and be sound:
'Twill hurt, but there are salves to friend you,
And many a balsam grows on ground.
And if your hand or foot offend you,
Cut it off, lad, and be whole;
But play the man, stand up and end you,
When the sickness is your soul.

—A. E. Housman, *A Shropshire Lad*, xlv.

The notion of suicide is invested with an awful grandeur in most people's minds. The sheer irrevocability of the act, the final plunge that tumbles the self-murderer into that shadowy realm "from which no traveler returns," strikes our hearts with gloomy solemnity. In Western culture the approaches to suicide are guarded with grim religious anathemas and barred by the threat of perpetual curses and soul-blasting bolts of spiritual lightning. Dante consigns suicides to the seventh circle of his Inferno, where their shades are transformed to trees in a dark forest whose bleeding branches are forever torn by demonic birds. Strict Christian dogma forbids the self-slain body to rest in hallowed ground. The monks who bury Ophelia, Hamlet's drowned sweetheart in Shakespeare's tragedy, allow her coffin into the churchyard only reluctantly, at the "great command" of the king. Otherwise, "she should in ground unsanctified have lodg'd, till the last trumpet."

Suicide has the power to unsettle us all, to make even the dullest brain philosophize for a few minutes about the meaning of life. It seems we alone of earth's creatures know we shall die. "Man has an angel's brain, and sees the axe from the first," writes the poet Edgar Lee Masters. From seeing the ax, to grasping the ax, to wielding the ax is a process that can occupy less than a minute, and there are actually cases, within the range of my experience, of wretches who chopped themselves to death with axes.

History is filled with heroic suicides: Cato the Younger falling on his sword at Utica, in North Africa, in 46 B.C., after having lost the last battle to save Rome's democracy, spending the whole night reading Plato's *Phaedo*, the dialogue on the immortality of the soul; the boy who "stood on the burning deck" of the French flagship *L'Orient*, at the battle of Aboukir Bay in 1798, and perished rather than abandon the body of the admiral, his father; the Buddhist monk, Thich Quang Duc, who immolated himself with gasoline in Saigon in 1963, to protest the corrupt regime of South Vietnam. These noble deaths resonate in human memory like a grand sculpture gallery of the mind. In our own days I have known of altruistic suicides, men who killed themselves out of kindness to others, in hopes of getting insurance settlements for their relatives, or as a means of liquidating debts. Nor is our own profession proof against the cumulative weight of doubt and pain that leads to self-murder. The renowned British forensic pathologist, Sir Bernard Spilsbury (1877–1947), took his own life after careful forethought. Having suffered several strokes, keenly aware that his mental acuity was impaired and that his professional usefulness was nearly at an end, Spilsbury made a significant gesture. He requisitioned only a hundred autopsy forms, instead of his usual five hundred. Day by day, the dead passed through his office, each case ticking off his self-allotted time. When the hundredth form was filled out, Spilsbury dined at his club, returned to his laboratory and gassed himself by placing his head in an oven.

Alas, my own experiences with suicides have usually taken me to ignobler places. What I see tends to be either rotten, or ridiculous, or simply sad. I am speaking here primarily of young people who commit suicide. I firmly believe that, if more would-be young suicides knew what grim jokes policemen will make about them, how unlovely a picture they will present to the technicians who must drag them away, autopsy them and compose their remains for burial, much of the imagined flash and glamour of the act of self-annihilation would evaporate. In most cases I have dealt with, suicide has proved to be a hasty, profligate, wasteful and ill-considered solution to a doubtful problem—a love thwarted, a reputation besmirched, a bank account overdrawn, a sudden temper tantrum or a drug-darkened depression. I do not include among these spur-of-the-moment extinctions the self-inflicted deaths of the terminally ill, for whom life has become a bitter and unsupportable burden. Loneliness, old age, incurable and painful illnesses, these are sometimes sufficient reasons for suicide. In such cases we ought to take a step backward, suspend judgment, and look with mercy upon those for whom death was a mercy.

Gallows humor and graveyard whistling are normal human reactions in the face of death. How many times have I heard police investigators, when confronted with a body that has four or five gunshot wounds to the head, or with its skull horribly crushed, or wrapped thickly with chains in a sunken, stove-in boat, say with mock solemnity: "Must be suicide, eh, Doc?"

And one cannot be too quick to disagree! Often suicides present the most bizarre injuries. When I was a graduate student, moonlighting in a hospital in Austin, I saw a truly extraordinary case: an attorney had committed suicide by shooting himself *five times* in the head with a .38 special at his desk, while his frantic secretary hammered at the locked door of his office! The door had been locked from the inside; there was no suspicion of the secretary's complicity in his death. The lawyer had acted entirely alone. When the police came to the room and took the gun from his hand, the wounded man was still very much alive, still able to look at them, follow them with his eyes. The shooting occurred late in the afternoon and it was my duty at the hospital to remain with him, during a painfully slow death watch, until he died at last, sometime after midnight. The investigation revealed that the unfortunate attorney had put the barrel of the gun in his mouth and fired five times. Two bullets had exited from the side of his face, two more exited his cranial vault near the top of the skull, and the fifth bullet remained lodged in his brain. It is not unusual for autopsies to disclose multiple gunshot wounds in suicide victims, although these occur most commonly in wounds of the torso. For a man to shoot himself five times in the head, and live as long as this lawyer did, was rare indeed.

Most suicides are far better thought out than most pregnancies. A tremendous deliberation, a dreadful persistence mark some of the self-inflicted deaths I have seen. In such cases the will to die can be as strong—even far stronger—than the will to live. Some suicide victims are willing to pass through hellish torments in order to attain the surcease from sorrow they crave. There is one case in the scientific literature in which a man managed to cut himself in two at the waist with a table saw. In old Japan, most cases of suicide committed by courtiers, called seppuku, involved slitting the stomach open with a sharp knife, after which the agony would be cut short by a friend who would step up and slit the dying man's throat. But there are other examples, notably that of the famous Marshal Maresuke Nogi in 1912, in which no accomplice was used, no coup de grâce was given. The victim quietly and stoically bled to death from the self-inflicted belly wound. One terrible case, published in the literature of our discipline, involved a man who wedged a large knife into an old radiator inside a church, then charged the knife repeatedly, butting the point with his head, until at last the blade pierced his skull and he died. Other documented cases have involved men who have killed themselves by raising the hydraulic tailgates of semi trucks, or lowering the raised beds of dump trucks, onto their necks and heads, like slow, blunt guillotines. In these cases the force of the machine-driven tailgate all but cuts the neck in two, mashing it to the consistency of a flattened noodle. There are also documented suicides by people who used chain saws on themselves, or purposely permitted themselves to be bitten to death by poisonous snakes.

There is a second type of suicide, which may be called the fastidious suicide, involving a person who wishes to look beautiful in death, to die tidily, or to cause as little trouble as possible to the investigators afterward. One case I recall involved a man who shot himself in the stomach twice, but was careful to position the barrel of the gun the second time so that the bullet entered exactly the same hole made by the first bullet. For some reason he did not want two entrance wounds in his stomach.

Women will often put on a pretty nightgown and apply makeup before killing themselves. One remarkable case in Ohio involved an eighteen-year-old girl who managed to shoot herself in the back by holding the revolver behind herself and pulling the trigger with her thumb. Her body revealed a single gunshot wound in the middle of her shoulder blades and at first glance the death looked like murder. But the angle of the limbs, the trajectory of the bullet and the fact that it took place in a room locked from the inside led police to realize it was suicide. Apparently the young woman was anxious to avoid disfiguring herself with a gunshot wound, so she would look nice in her casket.

Something similar occurred in a case of mine involving a dead man found in the Ocala National Forest. The corpse was found about fifty yards off the road, in the woods. All that remained when the body was located was a skeleton. Judging from the position of the skeleton, the man had apparently been seated, his back propped against a tree. Nearby was found a toiletries kit, including a can of pump-type toothpaste, aftershave, a container of Right Guard deodorant, nail clippers and razor blades, all contained neatly in an Adidas bag. The skeleton wore Adidas shoes and Dockers trousers. A ballpoint pen was found near his hand, but if he had written a note with it, the paper had long since disappeared. A bullet had pierced the skull, from one side to the other.

Everything about this solitary, seated skeleton in that lonely wood seemed to point to suicide—except for the fact that there was no gun! A zippered gun case was found right next to the body, but it was empty and the weapon was nowhere in sight. It stretched belief to imagine that a killer would shoot someone, take the murder weapon with him and leave the gun case behind. Where was the gun?

We searched for the better part of two days, using metal detectors, rakes and other tools, all around the tree where the skeleton had been found. Just before dusk on the second day, as I was moving leaves under a low bush with my trowel, I heard the clink of metal on metal: there, hidden by fallen leaves, was a .38-caliber snub-nosed revolver, about ten feet from the body. It was clearly the weapon used in the shooting.

But how did the gun get over there? Did someone come along, pick it up, see that it had begun to rust and then pitch it away? Was it dragged away by an animal eating part of the hand during decomposition? Such are the baffling questions that confront the forensic anthropologist. Nor was the young man ever identified. Somewhere in this country there may be parents who are still wondering about the fate of a perhaps troubled man in his early twenties, who went to Florida, walked into a deep forest and never walked out again. In a heroic effort to identify the remains, the police even investigated the manufacturing dates of the pump toothpaste, but to no avail. The gun used was a .38 Special made by Charter Firearms, and the police traced it to San Francisco, where it had been sold five years earlier. But the paper trail of the gun ended at that point.

Another interesting, meticulously planned suicide happened here in Gainesville a few years ago. It involved an instructor at the University of Florida who carefully taped a beer can opener and another metal object to his arm, wrapped the two frayed, bare ends of an electrical cord around these, plugged the cord into an appliance timer and set the timer to go off at 4 A.M. The man then took a large dose of sleeping pills, washed them down with whiskey and went calmly to bed. He slept soundly and never awakened. The appliance timer, electronically precise, completed its circuit at precisely 4 A.M. and electrocuted him, just as he had planned.

Another please-don't-fuss-over-me suicide in Gainesville involved a man who was found dead and decomposing in the front seat of his car, a hose leading from the exhaust through the cracked window on the driver's side. The car was out of gas, but the key in the ignition was switched to the running position. This was a straightforward case of carbon monoxide poisoning. The deceased left no note, but placed neatly alongside his body, on the seat of the car, was a business card belonging to Pete Zeller, the investigator in our local medical examiner's office. Pete was shocked to learn of this detail, and even more shocked to realize that he *knew* the dead man. He was an old acquaintance whom Pete had seen a couple of months earlier. The man had seemed in good spirits. Pete told the man he was now retired from the police and was working for the medical examiner's office. The man seemed fascinated by this information. He asked Pete casually what the best way of committing suicide might be. Just as casually, Pete answered that he believed carbon monoxide poisoning was relatively painless.

As the man said good-bye, Pete gave him one of his business cards, never dreaming of the use it would be put to. The man killed himself shortly afterward. He left Pete's card on the front seat as a kind of forwarding address, to make sure his remains would be properly taken care of. Pete had to endure some ribbing from his co-workers. "Pete," they said, "next time tell your suicidal friends to park their cars right outside the medical examiner's office. That way it saves us gasoline."

Many people, of course, kill themselves without meaning to. Accidental and natural deaths are often confused with suicides and murders. Very often an elderly person will fall, either down a flight of stairs, or in a bathroom, or someplace else, and the fall will produce lacerations and hemorrhages so severe that a careless observer might conclude the deceased had been bludgeoned to death. Such cases call for all the forensic pathologist's skill.

I know of one remarkable case in which a young man killed himself utterly by accident after he dressed himself up as a vampire, to go to a Halloween party. He wore a shirt stained with fake bloodstains, and beneath the shirt he had placed the end panel of a wooden apple crate, made of soft pine. As a final touch, for gory effect, he planned to appear at the party with a "stake" driven into his own heart. The stake would be transfixed in the soft pine panel underneath his shirt. Unfortunately, things did not work out as planned. The youth opted to use a sharp-pointed knife in lieu of a stake, and to tap the knife into the pine panel with a hammer. Obviously he believed the hidden wooden crate panel would shield him from harm. It didn't. The soft wood split easily beneath the hammer-driven knife point, and the blade plunged deep into the young man's heart. His last words, as he staggered out of his room, were a gasp of disbelief: "I really did it!" Then he toppled forward, dead. This was no true suicide, but instead an absurd and tragic accident.

But accidental self-inflicted deaths can spring from darker roots. In these deaths a certain type of aberrant sexual behavior reaches a different climax than that expected. I am referring to autoerotic asphyxiation.

This practice is very old, and very dangerous. In his perverse 1791 novel, *Justine,* the Marquis De Sade describes a French nobleman who is in the habit of hanging himself nearly to death, to enhance the intensity of orgasm during masturbation by restricting the flow of oxygen to his brain. By slow degrees, over a period of months, the nobleman increases the duration of the torture and the tightness of the noose, until at last he kills himself. Sade was a keen and clinical observer of aberrant behavior—not least his own—and people would do well to heed this cautionary tale. Sad to relate, this bizarre practice still flourishes today and is a well-recognized pattern of deviant behavior, one that often leads to disastrous results.

Whether this self-torture "works," whether there really is an intensification of sexual sensation in an oxygen-starved brain, or whether it is merely a ritualistic reenactment of execution fantasies or other sadomasochistic acts, I leave to the pathologists and the psychiatrists. What I do know, and what all of us who see these cases know, is that such behavior, once begun, goes from peak to peak and becomes increasingly dangerous the more it is practiced. And the strangulation ritual tends to be repeated, over and over again, over considerable periods of time. We know this because the beam, or pipe, or other solid object used to attach the other end of the rope is often found worn into a groove by long repetition of this activity.

Typically, the victim will knot a rope over a wooden beam, or a pipe in the basement, or a tree limb. He will then tie the other end of the rope around his neck, usually padding the neck with a towel or other materials to avoid rope burns or chafes. The hands may also be tied, usually with some sort of fast-release slip knot. Very often the victim is cross-dressed with panty hose and other items of women's attire. Often, too, explicit photographic pornographic material will be found on the floor near the victim.

Those who indulge in these perilous high jinks are courting death. They believe they can stop at any moment, but what they do not realize is that the inhibition of oxygen to the brain can cause the loss of consciousness *at any second, without any warning.* No one sends the man in the noose a telegram saying: "Your brain is about to shut down." And so they suddenly slump, inert, and then the constriction is intensified. Suffocation, asphyxiation without regaining consciousness, occurs in a matter of seconds. The victim will be found dead, in circumstances that would be excruciatingly embarrassing to him, if he were yet alive to see himself.

In the past, before this aberrant behavior was well documented, many of these cases were treated as homicides and suicides, instead of accidents. But crime marches on: murderers have learned this obscure wrinkle in human behavior and now attempt to set up false autoerotic asphyxiation scenes to throw investigators off the scent. In such cases, the presence or absence of the repetitive groove in the overhead beam can be all-important. Investigators will take note, too, of the fact that almost all practitioners of autoerotic asphyxiation are white males. No one knows why, but this is a statistical fact.

Nor are these deaths unusual. There is probably an average of one a month in my state, Florida. Occasionally we see some truly bizarre cases. Some men, literally afraid to risk their necks, have wrapped chains around their *waists* to cut off their breathing. This method of constriction is also effective in depriving the brain of oxygen. The victims then haul themselves aloft with chain hoists—from which they are later found dangling and dead. One wretch apparently enjoyed having his Volkswagen Beetle pull him slowly around with a chain wrapped about his waist. Unfortunately the chain got wrapped around a wheel and the car reeled him in, thrashing like a giant marlin, until he was crushed.

Another poor soul, for whom pain and pleasure were obviously closely akin, attached an electric train transformer to his penis with alligator clips and was in the habit of administering mild shocks to his genitals. Regrettably, on one occasion—the last!—the transformer shorted out, and he received the full 110-volt household electrical charge. He was instantly and ignominiously electrocuted. This case, when presented at one of our meetings, was interesting because the parents of the deceased had removed all evidence of the transformer before the police investigators showed up. They were understandably horrified and chagrined to discover their son dead under such sordid circumstances and did their best to conceal the manner of his death. But alligator clips leave very characteristic marks and these were plainly visible at the autopsy. After a few shrewd, discreet questions on the part of investigators, the unhappy parents broke down and revealed the full, shabby truth of the matter. The death was ruled accidental.

Milton Helprin, longtime chief medical examiner in New York City, used to tell the story of a young Irishman seen standing on the far reaches of a subway platform by several witnesses. At a certain point he suddenly and silently pitched forward right in front of an oncoming train. He was found dead beneath the wheels, horribly mangled. But his family was Catholic and did not readily accept the initial conclusion of suicide. They were quite certain their son had no reason to commit suicide, and in the end they were proved right. Helprin reexamined the mangled body and noticed tiny burn marks on the right thumb, index finger and the tip of the penis. He was able to reassure the family their son had died accidentally. He had been urinating on the subway tracks, and the stream had accidentally reached the third rail. The arc of falling water, rich with salts favoring conduction, instantly became an arc of lethal electricity. The lad was probably dead before he hit the tracks.

Of all the deaths I am called upon to investigate, suicides are among the most frustrating. Bones are my province, and most methods of suicide leave no evidence upon the skeleton. When we find a skeleton in the woods, fallen apart or disarticulated, I immediately look up, scanning the tree limbs above the skeleton, searching for some long-forgotten noose. As decomposition takes place in a hanging victim, the neck begins to stretch, until it may be several feet long. Finally the drying, mummifying skin will tear, head and trunk part company, and all falls down to earth, sundered in twain. The noose, however, may survive and point its hempen finger down at the truth.

Many of the skeletons that come to my laboratory belong to suicide victims who behaved like shy hermits in their final hours. Usually they are found in remote, out-of-the-way places. People often go to some hidden place to kill themselves, whether from a desire to act alone and unhindered, or because they wish simply to disappear in solitude, spending their last moments in reflective silence. In any event, by the time many of these bodies are found they are badly decomposed, perhaps only skeletons. It's up to us, the anthropologists, the pathologists, the investigators, to try to establish how these people came to die in such a secluded, pathless place. Inevitably these suicides get confused with straightforward murder victims who have been dumped in hidden locations. Another possibility is accidental death—the skeleton may belong to someone who took a drug overdose by mistake.

In cases involving poison or drugs, we always look for the pill bottles or the containers. Of course, many skeletons in the woods have a bottle with them—but it most likely contains a few remaining drops of Mad Dog 20-20, a potent, cheap wine. Such cases do indeed involve poisoning, the long slow poisoning of alcohol; but these deaths are not defined by law as suicidal.

But what if the victim took the drugs or the poison *before* going to the death scene? What if the poison was contained in a single capsule? In these cases, obviously, there won't be any evidence at the scene. Sometimes it happens that the victim flings the bottle away in horror or disgust after swallowing its contents. Such bottles are awfully difficult to find. In fact, I had one startling case involving a body found in the woods. In this case the police did a scene investigation and did not notice *two other* decomposing bodies fifty feet away. If you can miss a rotting corpse, imagine how easy it is to overlook a tiny pill bottle! The initial body was ruled not a suicide.

One would think that, when guns are involved in a suicide, the investigation would be a fairly straightforward matter. There's a hole in the head, a gun lying alongside the remains. Get the deceased identified, find a history of despondency—case closed! But in fact it doesn't work that way. The gun may be gone. A lot of people, happening on a body in the woods with a gun nearby, take the gun and leave the body unreported. Guns are valuable. And so the suicide, minus its gun, masquerades as murder and causes us no end of bother.

I have never encountered a note with the skeleton of a suicide. After remains have spent weeks or months in the wild, we count ourselves lucky indeed to find anything decipherable left on paper or plastic in these cases. Occasionally we'll get a telephone number on a matchbook cover or some other tiny clue, but not very often. The enormous Meek-Jennings suicide note, quoted elsewhere in this book, was the longest and most complex document of its kind ever to come before my eyes.

Euthanasia is legal in the Netherlands, and I can certainly understand suicide in the context of a terminal, incurable illness, when pain is great and insupportable or medical bills are accumulating ruinously. But most of the suicides I see seem to involve a lashing out, a last infliction of pain upon one's loved ones or family. All too often it's a boyfriend or girlfriend who blows his or her brains out in front of the person who has rejected them. These are hot-tempered acts of vengeance in which one's own death becomes a weapon meant to wound forever. Such cases often follow a curious etiquette, as though death were a last fling, a chance to go shopping. Sometimes we find the receipt from the gun store, where the weapon was bought a few days or hours earlier, even though it is quite rare for people to buy guns specifically to commit immediate suicide. Some of these weapons are extremely expensive, and the ammunition used is costly and sophisticated. And very often this last, lethal extravagance will be paid for with a credit card, because the new owner knows he won't be around to settle the bill. Charles Whitman, the mass murderer who killed sixteen people from his perch atop the famous tower at the University of Texas in 1966, used a rubber check to buy one of his weapons at Davis Hardware in Austin. The other he paid for with his Sears credit card.

The state of Florida has an inordinate number of suicides, particularly of the elderly. Over and over again, the same scenario unfolds: Mom and Pop, up in the Midwest, decide it is time to retire and go live the good life in sunny Florida. They little realize what pain awaits them! A year or two after moving into the trailer or condominium, Pop suffers a heart attack and Mom is left alone, or vice versa. Every living soul the survivor knows is back home in the Midwest. To return or stay? Somehow going back seems harder than going forward. The survivor hangs on in Florida, but the sands of life are ebbing away. Gradually there is a sinking, a submersion into a sea of strangers. The long, sunny days become painful and tedious; all seems overbright and irritating in these hot latitudes. Suicide becomes a soothing way out of a painful, empty existence.

I sometimes wish, as Florida fills up with refugees from the northern United States, that we could put brutally honest signs up at the state borders. "SENIORS! WELCOME TO FLORIDA!" they would say.

"BE ADVISED YOU ARE NOT JUST LEAVING THE SNOWS BEHIND; YOU ARE LEAVING YOUR LIVES BEHIND." People who come to Florida all too often do not realize how painful our peculiar rootless newness can be. Naples, Fort Myers, St. Petersburg, Miami Beach—these communities sit atop invisible cliffs, overlooking abysses of self-extinction for the elderly.

One such case, memorable to me chiefly because of the dead man's teeth, involved a skeletonized set of remains found in Polk County, near Disney World, in 1987. He had a bullet hole in the center of his skull and a gun lying beside him. He also had a perfect set of teeth, not particularly worn, with no fillings and not a single cavity. His teeth were as unmarred as a child's, but fully grown and in the mouth of an adult. The medical examiner called me from his district in central Florida and wanted to know the age of the remains. He estimated the deceased was in his forties, primarily because of these flawless teeth. I looked at the skeleton, especially at the spinal column, and said the man was older than sixty-five years of age, probably older than seventy.

I think the medical examiner concealed a polite smile at the apparent absurdity of my findings. But I stuck to my findings. I can't always be right but I have to say what I have concluded. Without much confidence, he passed on my findings to the police, who began to investigate further. Almost immediately they verified that the very gun found with the body had been sold to an eighty-year-old man who had been missing for several months. When the man's dental records were checked, those extraordinary, perfect teeth shone forth intact from the x-ray light table. For a lucky handful of people in this world there is no such thing as tooth decay. Their teeth naturally resist all cavities, and normal wearing away is replaced by upwellings of dentin, the inner material of the tooth, rising and replacing the worn enamel like tiny fountains of youth. This old gentleman was among these happy few, but he was unhappy nonetheless. Neighbors confirmed that he had been acting despondent before he disappeared. The rest of the puzzle pieces fell into place easily. Age was all, in this case. When the police began looking for an eighty-year-old instead of a forty-year-old, the matter was quickly solved.

After exercising our wits to their utmost, we investigators sometimes have to confess failure. Killing is killing, whether it be directed against oneself or another, and in some cases it is simply impossible to decide whether a victim died by his own hand or someone else's. *"You killed him and then made it look like suicide!"* is more than a hackneyed line from the movies. Sometimes it comes true.

I remember a notorious crack house that burned down in Jacksonville some years ago. The incinerated remains of a young woman were found in the smoldering ruins. At first she was thought by police to have perished in the fire. When I examined her closely, however, I saw there were burned maggots on the body—clear evidence she had been dead and decomposing at least forty-eight to seventy-two hours before the fire. Was she a homicide victim? Had she died of a drug overdose? Had she committed suicide? I cannot tell. No one can tell. The nameless burned woman remains one of the many enigmas in my career. I wish that every case had an answer, but it seems that questions always outnumber answers in my world.

Outpacing the Fiend

Like one, that on a lonesome road
Doth walk in fear and dread,
And having once turned round, walks on,
And turns no more his head;
Because he knows a frightful fiend
Doth close behind him tread. . . .

—Samuel Taylor Coleridge,
The Rime of the Ancient Mariner

We forensic anthropologists owe a dark debt to murderers. From the beginning, our science has walked almost abreast of homicide, trying to outpace the "frightful fiend" who commits it. Sometimes we are scarcely half a step ahead; sometimes we are several steps behind. In all such cases our instructors are assassins. It is our task to solve—or at least try to solve—terrible problems put before us by men who have slain their fellow men. Over the years, these brutal teachers have brought out the best in us, stimulated us, put us on our mettle. By challenging us to unravel seemingly impossible knots of malevolence, the killers have ultimately helped us in the advancement of science and the spread of knowledge. It is a singular fact that some of the most dazzling pieces of detective work in our profession have come about as a direct result of some extraordinarily depraved murder. The darker the crime, the brighter shines the solution.

Ours is a remarkably new science. Accurate bone measurement began only in 1755, when Jean Joseph Sue (1710–92), an anatomy professor at the Louvre, published the complete measurements of four bodies and the maximum lengths of many of the bones of fourteen cadavers ranging in age from a six-week-old fetus to an adult of twenty-five years. From these late beginnings, and from a handful of interesting cases, a broad field of forensic investigation has come into being, so wide, so active, so thriving today that we hold annual conventions at which hundreds of forensic scientists meet to delve into a panoply of cases, old and new. It is a field in which Americans can claim noteworthy achievements—both in crime and in its subsequent investigation.

Here in America the science of forensic anthropology can trace its origins directly to a celebrated murder, that of Dr. George Parkman, killed in 1849 by a Harvard professor who owed him money. Parkman's murder was investigated by another Harvard professor, Oliver Wendell Holmes. Both men had sons who would be more famous than their fathers. Parkman's was Francis Parkman, who became one of America's greatest historians, and whose *Oregon Trail* has become a classic. Holmes's son would later serve with distinction in the Civil War, in which he was thrice wounded, and would go on to become one of America's greatest Supreme Court justices, dying only in 1935.

At the time of the murder the elder Holmes held the Parkman professorship of anatomy, endowed by and named after George Parkman himself. So in a way Parkman reached out from the grave and helped bring his own murderer to justice.

Parkman was a wealthy Boston physician and landlord who donated the land where Harvard Medical School now stands. Vain, a notorious skinflint, he ordered new dentures to wear at the groundbreaking ceremony for the medical school and told his dentist, Dr.

Nathan Keep, that if the new false teeth couldn't be finished in time for the ceremony he wouldn't pay a cent for them. Working frenziedly, Dr. Keep just managed to finish the dentures in time, and luckily kept the mold of Parkman's jaw, which he had used to model the teeth.

In the meantime the avaricious Parkman had lent a sum of money to a Harvard anatomy professor named John Webster. When Parkman dunned Webster for the repayment of this loan, Webster murdered him, dismembered his body and hid pieces of it among other remains in his anatomy laboratory, where it was unlikely to arouse suspicion. The rest of the corpse Webster concealed in his indoor privy, where the pieces were found by a suspicious janitor, who broke through a wall to discover them. Other bits of the doctor's body, including his lower jaw, were found burned in an assayer's furnace nearby.

The police at first detained the janitor, believing he had committed the murder. Close scrutiny of Parkman's scattered remains in the laboratory by Holmes and his colleague, anatomist Jeffries Wyman, revealed that the remains in question were not anatomical lab specimens—they had not been treated with any preserving chemicals. They all came from the same body, and that body belonged to a man fifty to sixty years old who stood about five feet ten inches tall (Parkman was fifty and stood five-ten). Finally, the false teeth retrieved from the bed of the assaying furnace perfectly fit the model of Parkman's jaw that Keep had kept.

Confronted with this evidence, the guilty Webster finally broke down and confessed that he had killed Parkman "in a fit of rage." Webster was tried, convicted and hanged for the murder in 1850.

The Parkman case received tremendous publicity at the time and probably influenced young Thomas Dwight (1843–1911), then only a boy of seven, to devote his career to the study of anatomy. Today Dwight is honored as the father of American forensic anthropology. A Bostonian, Dwight spent nearly forty years as an investigator and teacher of anatomy, and during the last twenty-eight years of his career he held the Parkman professorship of anatomy at Harvard. Throughout his life Dwight published papers on skeletons, their identification and differentiation by sex, age and height. An essay of his in 1878 was the first of its kind in this field.

Dwight's most famous pupil was George A. Dorsey (1868–1931), a multitalented man who was interested in ethnology, photography and, almost as a sideline, the human skeleton. Dorsey's career, too, was given a huge boost by a notorious murder that he helped solve, the gruesome case of the Chicago sausage maker, Adolph Luetgert.

Luetgert murdered his wife Louisa in 1897. Since he ran a sausage factory, he was in a unique position to make her body disappear. Louisa Luetgert was murdered at home, but her husband transported her body in a carriage by night to his five-story factory at the corner of Diversey and Hermitage streets in Chicago. There he plunged it into a huge vat filled with a caustic solution containing 375 pounds of potash. Evidence later brought out at his trial indicated that Luetgert sat beside the vat stirring the grisly mixture all through the night. In the morning he was found sleeping in his office, with the vat overflowing and a greasy substance all over the floor. The acidic potash had leached out most of the calcium from Louisa Luetgert's bones, gradually reducing them to jelly. This was the "grease" noticed the next morning on the floor.

Luetgert reported his wife missing, but after a few days her brother began to suspect foul play. A search of the factory by police yielded Louisa Luetgert's ring and four tiny pieces of human bone in congealed sediment in the vat, which had by then been drained. Luetgert was charged with his wife's murder. His defense was bold and straightforward: there was no *corpus delicti*. Louisa Luetgert's body had been dissolved.

But in one of the most brilliant courtroom displays of forensic anthropology ever witnessed, George Dorsey was able to prove that the four tiny fragments of bone, so small that all four of them together would fit on a silver quarter dollar, were parts of a human skeleton. The bones introduced in evidence were: the end of a metacarpal from the hand, a head of a rib, a portion of a phalanx, or toebone, and a sesamoid bone from the foot. These minuscule fragments, together with Louisa Luetgert's ring, were enough to convict Adolph Luetgert and send him to prison for life. Even though Luetgert had not attempted to convert his wife to sausage, the memory of the case gave the factory such a bad name that it was soon forced to shut down for lack of business. Dorsey in 1898 published a landmark paper, "The Skeleton in Medico-Legal Anatomy," based on his research in the Luetgert case.

After this extraordinary coup, however, Dorsey gave up anatomy and devoted himself to the study and photography of North American Indians. He later became the U.S. naval attaché in Spain. In those days forensic anthropology was not recognized as a science but only as a subbranch of anatomy that could occasionally furnish interesting information to the police.

One of the rarest and most interesting books in my library is a black and gold volume called *Medico-Legal Aspects of the Ruxton Case*, published in 1937. Written by John Glaister, M.D., and James Couper Brash, M.D., this remarkable book examines, with amazing detail and thoroughness, one of the most grisly and notorious double murders committed in this century. These murders, moreover, were carried out by a doctor with a good knowledge of anatomy, who was determined to destroy all evidence of his crime. The Ruxton case is probably the single most quoted murder discussed in modern forensic textbooks.

This weird and grisly double killing has a rich, period flavor of England about it. British society in the mid-1930s emerges from Glaister and Brash's account as so remarkable, cohesive and tightly interdependent that one wonders how anybody ever got away with murder at all.

Witnesses abound in the Ruxton case. People knock at his door all day long while the murderer is about his gruesome task of dismembering the bodies. Charwomen later recall horrible odors and strange stains. A bandage on the doctor's finger arouses a neighbor's suspicion. The killer rents a car to dispose of the bodies and promptly collides with a bicyclist, who calls the police, who make a full report. The entire British press is in full cry against the criminal.

Brilliant specialists step forward to reconstruct the remains in detail, matching their reconstructions with known photographs of the victims. The hapless murderer is arrested, pleads he is innocent—in vain. Surrounded by eyes that see all, ears that hear the least whisper, memories that let nothing slip, pursued by vigilant constables on bicycles and by sober cleaning ladies, the culprit is overwhelmed by the evidence, found guilty, and hanged. The majesty of British law triumphs absolutely. It is interesting to speculate what effect the Ruxton case may have had upon the young film director, Alfred Hitchcock, who was just then coming into his own in Great Britain. In Hitchcock's movies, murder will out, always. No one escapes punishment. The police are omnipotent and omniscient figures of dread.

Dr. Buck Ruxton was born in 1899 in India. He was a Parsee whose real name was Bikhtyar Rostomji Ratanji Hakim ("Hakim" means "doctor"), and he took his Bachelor of Medicine degrees at Bombay and London universities. After settling in England, Ruxton took a mistress, Isabella Van Ess, whom he described to neighbors as his wife. The couple lived in Lancaster and had a stormy relationship. "We were the kind of people who could not live with each other and could not live without each other," Ruxton later told police. The pair fought frequently and twice Mrs. Ruxton sought police protection.

On September 7, 1935, Ruxton accused his wife of having an affair with the Lancaster town clerk. Soon after this she disappeared. Isabella was last seen alive on Saturday, September 14, at 11:30 A.M. On Sunday the doctor paid a visit to his charwoman, Agnes Oxley, who was scheduled to come clean the house on Monday morning at seven-fifteen. He asked Oxley not to come Monday, but instead on Tuesday. He explained that his wife was away on a holiday to Edinburgh.

On Monday, September 16, several tradesmen and one patient called at Ruxton's house at 2 Dalton Square. They were all turned away. Ruxton explained that he was busy redoing the carpets in the house and showed the would-be patients his hands: "Look how dirty they are," he said. To one of these visitors Ruxton said that his wife's personal maid, Mary Rogerson, had gone with her to Scotland on the same holiday.

At 11:30 A.M. that same day Ruxton took his children to a friend's house, asking him to look after them. The friend noticed Ruxton's finger was cut and bandaged. Ruxton explained he had cut it that morning, opening a can of peaches. One can only speculate about what he was really opening. Dismembering a human body is a very tricky procedure. I have had to do it myself, and, though I have never cut myself with a scalpel, I was once cut by another doctor's knife, when he lost control of it. I have also been cut by the sharp end of a broken bone that was floating around loose inside the torso of a plane crash victim.

Dr. Ruxton later went over to the maid's house and explained to her parents, the Rogersons, that their daughter was on vacation with his wife in Scotland and would not be back for a week or two.

That Monday afternoon Ruxton asked a patient of his, a Mrs. Hampshire, to come over to his house and scrub down the staircase. Mrs. Hampshire agreed. When she went into the bathroom, she noticed the tub was stained yellow and even a vigorous scouring with Vim cleanser could not remove the discoloration. Ruxton gave Mrs. Hampshire one of his suits, badly stained, as a present. "He said I could have it cleaned," she told police later. The next day Ruxton apparently changed his mind and asked for the suit back. When Mrs. Hampshire tried to clean the carpets, the scrubbing water turned blood-red.

On this same busy Monday, Ruxton rented a car and on Tuesday, September 17, he was involved in a slight collision with a cyclist at Kendal, in the Lake District. To a policeman investigating the accident, Ruxton said he was returning from a business trip in Carlisle.

The charwoman came as scheduled on September 17, letting herself into the empty house. Two other charwomen were brought in to clean the house as well, up to the day of September 20. All later complained of bad stains and odors in the house. Ruxton sent one of them to buy eau de Cologne and a sprayer, and the house was sprayed and fumigated.

On September 29 the dismembered remains of two women were found in a ravine near Moffat, Scotland. The bodies were so mutilated and decomposed that at first it was supposed that one of them belonged to a man. Ruxton, upon seeing the news in the newspaper, remarked to Mrs. Oxley: "So you see . . . it is not our two."

On October 9, Mary Rogerson's mother informed police that her daughter was missing. The next day Ruxton himself went to the police and asked that "discreet inquiries" be made "with a view to finding my wife."

A blouse and a pair of children's rompers belonging to Ruxton's children were found with the remains at Moffat (the rompers had been used to wrap one of the severed heads). The newspapers speculated openly about Ruxton's involvement and the doctor complained to the police that the publicity was "ruining my practice."

On October 13, Ruxton was charged with the murder of Mary Rogerson and on November 5 with that of Isabella. The police said Ruxton had murdered his wife and then killed the maid because she saw the murder or its immediate aftermath. The doctor pleaded not guilty and called the charges "absolute bunkum, with a capital B."

The remains found in the Scottish ravine consisted of two skulls, two torsos, seventeen parts of limbs and forty-three portions of soft tissue. All identifying characteristics had been carefully removed from the remains. One set of hands, later found to belong to Isabella Van Ess, was found with the fingertips cut off, to prevent fingerprinting. The other pair was left intact, presumably because the killer believed no fingerprints of Mary Rogerson were on file with the police. On the other hand, Mary Rogerson had had a squint in one eye, and the eyes from one skull had been carefully removed. By the same token, Mrs. Ruxton's legs had been noticeably fat and untapering down to the ankle—and the soft tissue from the legs of one body had been sliced away. Even a distinguishing bunion had been hacked off a severed foot. Both bodies had been dismembered and drained of blood after death.

Almost every conceivable point of scientific attack, every distinguishing characteristic that might have identified either of the two corpses, was foreseen, seized upon and obliterated by the murderer with diabolical thoroughness.

Yet in the end the bodies were identified beyond all question, in a brilliant process of forensic detection that is still a landmark today. Glaister and Brash reconstructed the bodies in the Ruxton affair, took photographs of the mutilated remains, posed them at certain angles, and compared them to photos of the two murder victims in life, taken at the selfsame angles. The resulting photographs are not for the faint of heart. In the final superimpositions, the mutilated skulls were ghosted into photographs of the victims taken when alive, and shine through them like silvery death's heads. This photographic evidence was devastating. The disfigured skulls agreed with the living portraits in every detail.

Dr. Buck Ruxton was tried, found guilty, sentenced to death and hanged at Strangeways Jail, Manchester, on May 21, 1936.

I was born the year after Ruxton was hanged. It often strikes me how relatively young our science of forensic anthropology is. With the exception of a handful of great, departed pioneers, I have seen and known personally many of the principal figures of our field. Indeed, many of them are still alive today.

Our discipline is so new fledged that even in the 1930s the recently founded FBI had to take its cases across the street to the Smithsonian Institution for analysis. There the Division of Physical Anthropology was led by a brilliant anatomist whose picture later appeared on a Czechoslovakian postage stamp: Aleš Hrdlička (pronounced "Hurd-LICH-ka"). Hrdlička had come to the Smithsonian in 1903. He was a remarkable, eccentric man, very slender, bald, mustached and proper. He invariably wore a high, starched collar and he was very tight-fisted. Colleagues still tell stories of how, on business trips, he would step up to the front desk of a hotel with a paper bag full of skulls and bones in one hand—the bones would be sticking out of the top of the bag—and a small valise in the other.

Then he would loudly request a room without a bath, to save money. Hrdlicka became founding editor of the *American Journal of Physical Anthropology* and is responsible for beginning the Smithsonian's vast collection of human skeletons, which today numbers over 33,000 specimens.

But Hrdliçka never published any of his cases. I suspect his greatest successes lie buried deep in FBI archives. He left pupils, admirers, colleagues who had learned much from him—but not a word to posterity. The science of forensic anthropology had to wait until 1939 for the appearance of a paper that summed up everything about the human skeleton known up to that time. This was Wilton Marion Krogman's *Guide to the Identification of Human Skeletal Material,* which was originally published not by any university or scholarly press but by the FBI. In 1958, Krogman published an expanded version of his paper in book form: *The Human Skeleton in Forensic Medicine,* which appeared just at the time I elected to enter the field. Krogman himself worked at the University of Pennsylvania and lived to be ninety-nine years old. He was active to the end, though he used to complain, just shy of a century, that his eyesight was failing!

One of my most distinguished colleagues, Dr. Ellis R. Kerley, propagated our discipline far and wide among other forensic scientists. I first met Ellis when I interviewed at the University of Kansas, around 1971. After I joined the American Academy of Forensic Sciences in 1974, I came to know him better. Ellis has been a mentor for many of us in the field, a very lovable man, the only forensic anthropologist ever to have served as president of the academy, and the man who pioneered the organization of our section within the academy. In a sense, we all rode in on Ellis's coattails. Ellis also worked with Dr. Lowell Levine and Clyde Snow on the identification of the remains of Dr. Josef Mengele, the Nazi "Angel of Death," who eluded justice after the war and finally drowned in Brazil in 1979. DNA samples from Mengele's surviving family members in Germany proved conclusively that the bones in a certain grave were his. Ellis was also called in to examine the remains of the astronauts who died in the *Challenger* space shuttle disaster in 1986. Because of the terrific force of the explosion and the subsequent long fall to the ocean, the remains were very fragmentary and immense pains were taken to ensure proper identification. Details of the condition of these remains have never been made public, but Ellis's reputation is so great that no one has ever dreamed of questioning them.

Krogman's brief *Guide* became the Bible of the new science, both for the FBI and for the United States Army, which soon had to deal with thousands of skeletonized dead American soldiers, sailors and airmen in World War II. The furious island battles in the Pacific Theater, and the back-and-forth fighting later on in Korea, resulted in many remains being left on the field to be retrieved later. Those without dogtags could only be gathered up by the Army Quartermaster Corps and taken to military mortuaries for identification. Often the skeletons of Japanese and Koreans were mixed in with the American remains, and it became a matter of some importance to separate our dead from these other bones of Asiatic origin. (Korea was the last American war in which large numbers of American dead were abandoned or buried on the battlefield. By the time of the Vietnam War, advances in mobility and transport enabled most American soldiers to be evacuated immediately from combat zones, whether they were wounded or dead.)

Partly because of the United States campaigns in the Pacific, the Central Identification Laboratory in Hawaii (CILHI) was set up in 1947. Charles E. Snow (1910–67) was the first physical anthropologist to serve there. Mildred Trotter, who is still with us today, was another. Trotter has won an extraordinary reputation in our field for her great contributions to anatomy and osteology. My own teacher, Tom McKern (1920–74), worked on these war dead in 1948–49. McKern collaborated with another well-known anthropologist, T. Dale Stewart, in identifying and measuring the remains of 450 skeletons of men killed in the Korean War.

Dale Stewart was a devoted disciple of Hrdlička's. He admired the old man so much that he painted a portrait of him and hung it in his office; and Hrdlička's ashes are in an urn next to the portrait. Dale himself was an extremely active, fit man who broke his hip while in his eighties and used to demonstrate how well it had healed by doing jumping jacks for anyone who cared to watch. He used to get into terrific scholarly arguments with another legendary figure in our field, Larry Angel. Larry was a Harvard-educated anthropologist, bald, with muttonchop whiskers and a brilliant, restless mind. I never heard Larry talk about anything but his work. It was a sight to behold, to see these two giants—giants in intellect, but men of very small physical stature—Stewart and Angel, quarreling loudly with each other at the Smithsonian over pubic symphyses (the pubic symphysis is a part of the skeleton which changes throughout life and can be crucial in determining age). Larry was an extraordinary character in his own right, a dazzling teacher who used to astonish police and FBI agents by *tasting* bone samples placed in front of him. It looked shocking enough, but there was a reason why Larry did what he did. Small fragments of bones often get mixed up with rocks, and it can be difficult to tell the two apart. But you can decide immediately whether a small lump of material is bone or rock by touching it to your tongue. Bone will stick to your tongue because of its porous nature. Rock will not. It is a trick I use myself, from time to time. But it does cause talk.

For us forensic anthropologists, 1973 is the year we came of age as a discipline. It was in that year that the new section of physical anthropology was established within the American Academy of Forensic Sciences, with fourteen members. This is our own section and we meet once a year at the academy's convention. Our work is published in the *Journal of Forensic Sciences,* and within its pages are articles with such titles as: "Injuries to Cadavers Resulting from Experimental Rear Impact" (an article for which six corpses were strapped into automobiles and test-crashed to see what postmortem trauma would look like); "The Effect of Severe Bedsores on Bone"; "The Individuality of Human Footprints"; and "The Mummified Heart."

I have not missed an academy convention since 1974, the year I joined, and I look forward to every reunion with intense anticipation. I love these meetings because they represent the only chance I get to see many of my colleagues—and many of my colleagues are extremely colorful people. The extraordinary Clyde Snow can be relied upon to tell hair-raising stories, in his Southwestern drawl, of the latest bodies he's examined in war zones in Bosnia, Afghanistan or Guatemala. Papers are presented on new research and techniques. The former New York City medical examiner, Dr. Michael Baden, hosts a "Bring Your Own Slides" evening, at which some truly astounding images are presented.

One of the highlights of our meetings is the proceedings of the Last Word Society, in which each participant will present a paper on some vexing historical problem. Among the riddles we have debated are these: Was Vincent Van Gogh's color imagery and style the result of digitalis poisoning? Did Charles Darwin suffer from nicotine toxins? Who was Jack the Ripper? Did King Richard III really order the murder of the two princes in the Tower of London? What was the final body count in the legendary crash that killed Notre Dame football coach Knute Rockne? What was the final body count in the legendary feud between the Hatfields and McCoys?

One comes away from the AAFS convention with renewed energy to try something new, do something differently. Perhaps we will exchange notes, reprints or case reports with each other. Perhaps we will feel encouraged to check an unidentified skeleton to see if it matches a missing person we've heard described during a meeting. Sometimes we bring specimens to the conventions, not to fool each other but in honest perplexity. We are baffled, so we solicit one another's opinions. Often the advice we get is invaluable. These annual meetings are a splendid opportunity for us to trade ideas, to scrape away the rust of academic isolation.

During these annual proceedings applicants who wish to become diplomates of the American Board of Forensic Anthropology are examined. Involved are two days of rigorous examination, a day of written tests, followed by a day of on-the-spot identification of skeletal specimens. The second day's exams obviously require the presence of the dead as well as the living, and some of us have to bring specimens of bones to the convention.

This requires some explanation, particularly at airports. I always make a point of telling the airline ticket agent just how many skulls I have with me in my baggage—not to shock her, but to make sure that, in case the plane crashes, investigators will know why there were more skulls than passengers aboard. This is mere professional courtesy to my colleagues, who will have to pick through my remains in the event of an accident.

Once, I recall, we were using the skeletal collections of a major museum for exam purposes. This museum had some very interesting specimens, including many samples of gunshot victims from the Texas Revolution in the early part of the nineteenth century. But the most fascinating skeleton in the bunch wasn't a victim of war, or murder, or any violent death. It was the skeleton of one of the curators of the museum, who had bequeathed his bones to the collection, where they had remained for many years. These bones stood out, not for any deep scientific reason, but because they had bits of tinsel still sticking to them.

Tinsel! We were told that this curator's skeleton had been "invited" to many Christmas parties at the museum in the years after his death. We also heard that his bones had been bedecked with Christmas decorations—and the evidence of the tinsel was sparkling, conclusive proof that the rumors were true. I am usually against lighthearted treatment of human remains, but in this case I suspended judgment. The man in life was loved. He left his bones to the museum where he had spent his happiest days. It was no very great wrong, I think, for his successors to take his bones to Christmas parties he would himself have enjoyed, alive. And if they saluted his memory with festive cups of eggnog, and decked his bones with tinsel and ornaments, they did so out of sincere respect and affection for a departed scientist. *That* is true camaraderie!

Unnatural Nature

In nature, there's no blemish but the mind;
None can be called deform'd, but the unkind.

—Shakespeare, *Twelfth Night,*
Act III, Scene 4

I have spent most of my life exploring the extraordinary proper-
ties of human bone and the close-knit harmony of the human skeleton. From the pale, translucent, pearly luster of the fetal skeleton, so
delicate and wraithlike, to the ghastly, disfiguring eruptions and out-
bubblings that seethe up like scorched milk from the extraordinary
bones of Joseph Merrick, the renowned "Elephant Man" of the
1880s, the mortal frame of the human body—the skeleton—is to me
an object of inexhaustible wonder, a book I shall never finish reading.

If there is one thing I have sought to impress on my students, it
is that they must not think of bones as solid and unchanging. The
astonishing hardness and durability of human bone can deceive the
untaught into thinking that bone is something rocklike and change-
less. Nothing could be further from the truth. Our skeletons are
constantly in flux, constantly reshaping themselves. While we live,
our bones are alive, formed of a swarm of living cells embedded and

surrounded in the matrix of the bone wall, basking in the warmth of the blood cells they create in their inmost marrow. The covering of the bone, the periosteum, is constantly spinning forth new bone cells, destroying old ones. Throughout our lives our bones change from one hour to the next. As we age, they begin slowly to fuse together, to remodel themselves, to grow stiffer, more brittle and less elastic. Nor am I exempted from this process simply because I have studied it in some detail: inside my own body, across autumns and winters, I sense the slow approach of age by the gradual, ineluctable stiffening of my joints. With each passing year, my movements are slightly more circumscribed. I am my skeleton's mask and puppet, as you are yours.

We keep no secrets from our bones. We blurt out everything shamelessly to these silent, obedient servants of our days. Within the archives of our skeletons are written down the intimate diaries of our lives: our ancestry, our illnesses, our injuries and infirmities, the patterns of our labor and exercise, sometimes even our most secret sins and blush-worthy abuses. All we have been, or nearly, is inscribed and enclosed in our skeletons, to be revealed at last when they stand forth naked, the flesh having fallen away from them. To read all of these things—that is the art of forensic anthropology.

Of what does this remarkable structure consist? The great English stylist and polymath, Sir Thomas Browne (1605–82), marveled that so little should be left of a man, after cremation:

> *How the bulk of a man should sink into so few pounds of bones and ashes, may seem strange unto any who considers not its constitution. . . . Even bones themselves reduced to ashes do abate a notable proportion. And consisting much of a volatile salt, when that is fired out, make a light kind of cinders. . . .*

Browne was a shrewd observer. Fire does indeed resolve bone into its two essential components: one that is inorganic and made up of minerals such as calcium carbonate, and the other consisting of more complex organic chemicals.

These organic portions of the bone include a material called collagen—you may know it from shampoo commercials on television. Collagen is a marvelous substance that gives bone its elasticity, adding to its strength and preventing breakage. It gives the bone the ability to bend and flex within tolerable limits. We would shatter at every fall, like china dolls, were it not for collagen. It is possible to leach the calcium and other inorganic chemicals out of a fresh bone by soaking it in a dilute solution of acid, such as hydrochloric acid. What remains after this acid bath is a specimen of what appears to be hard rubber. So elastic is the bone at this point that a fibula—the long thin bone from the lower portion of the leg—can sometimes carefully be tied into an overhand knot.

The disease osteomalacia—"bone-softness" in Greek—is characterized by a superabundance of collagen, disproportionate to the inorganic bone matrix. The victims of this disease are able to tie their legs in knots and perform other amazing and shocking contortions. Such prodigies formerly inhabited circus sideshows and were advertised as "The India-Rubber Man" or "The Boneless Wonder." The latter was mentioned by Winston Churchill in a famous parliamentary speech lampooning Prime Minister Ramsay MacDonald in 1931. As a youth, Churchill said, he had longed to see the Boneless Wonder in P. T. Barnum's circus, but he was forbidden to do so by his parents, "who judged that the spectacle would be too revolting and demoralizing for my youthful eyes.

"I have waited fifty years," Churchill said scathingly, while turning to face Ramsay MacDonald, "to see the Boneless Wonder sitting on the Treasury bench."

The other, inorganic component of bone is what remains after a fire or long action by the sun. All the organic compounds are volatized away and what is left is a chalky residue: "calcined bones." Here is bone at its driest, purged of all its organic compounds by heat. But diseases, too, can rob a bone of collagen and, when collagen departs, elasticity departs as well. Osteoporosis, hyperparathyroidism and *osteogenesis imperfecta*—all these conditions are essentially imbalances in bone chemistry, rendering bones brittle as twigs.

Sometimes children with these disorders are brought to hospital emergency rooms with one or more broken bones and are diagnosed as victims of child abuse. They aren't. Their bones, not their parents, are to blame.

One particularly horrific disease, *leontiasis ossea,* which is mercifully rare, causes huge foamy eruptions and effusions of bone, jutting up from the skull, forming horrid crowns and bubbles of bone. The skulls of the victims of this disease seem to start up in waves and combs, resembling a lion's shaggy mane.

All of us have seen the brain teaser in newspapers: how many bones are there in the human body? The answer is usually upward of two hundred, but the question is terribly unscientific. The number of bones in your body strictly depends on the time in your life you are talking about. Even after maturity it varies. The bones of the coccyx, the tailbone, will fuse together. In the bones of some adults the breastbone will be a single bone, but in others it is still two or three bones. In some older individuals you may find only a few dozen separate elements, because so many bones have fused together. There are even cases on record of skeletons being totally fused into a single solid mass. In such an extreme case, the individual must choose whether he wishes to spend the brief remainder of his life in a sitting or standing position.

The pangs of childbirth, the Bible says, are fleeting and immediately repaid by the joys of new motherhood. But women should know that a record of those days is etched permanently in the surface of their pelvises as "parturition scars." These scars begin to form in about the fourth month of pregnancy, when a hormone that softens the tendons that knit the pelvic bones together is released. To use a bit of shop talk, these telltale signs of childbirth appear on the dorsal side of the pubic symphysis near the margins of the articular surfaces and in the preauricular grooves or sulci of the ilia. In plain English, this means that women often carve notches in their pelvises after every childbirth, the way gunfighters in the American West carved notches in their pistol butts after every death.

Beauty is in the eye of the beholder, but I believe a case might be made that female skeletons are more beautiful than their male counterparts. There are actual scientific terms to distinguish the aesthetic impression a female skeleton makes, as opposed to a male. Such terms are aids to identification, or "sexing the skeleton," as we call it. A typical female set of bones is said to be *gracilis*—smoother, less knobbly, with edges gracefully planed or beveled, as if by an invisible adze. A typical male is *robustus*. His bones are thick, pitted and bumped with rough irregularities where the muscles and tendons were attached. These qualities of robustness and gracefulness are used in determining the sex of skeletons that are incomplete or immature, and they are often very subjective. There are bits of skeletons, especially those of children and adolescents, in which the sex distinction is obviously very blurry. Female body builders are creating knotty lumps on their bones where their hard-won new muscles are anchored, so their bones look more robust. Transsexual men who take estrogen are going in the opposite direction, moving from *robustus* to *gracilis*, making their skeletons smoother and more equivocal.

Certain it is that the female skull is visibly more polished and even-surfaced than the male skull, as if it had been turned on some invisible potter's wheel. We men are rough creatures, even in our inmost core. The male skull has a square jaw and heavy brows. We sport craggy bumps and knots and projections where our muscles are anchored. Our skulls often look as though they were sculpted of rough clay. The same is true of male arm and leg bones. Males have big knobby joints. If you don't believe it, go to the beach and look at the knees. The length of a person's hair may deceive you, but the knees—never!

One of the most puzzling cases I ever handled occurred over in Jacksonville some years ago. A completely dry and fleshless skeleton was found next to a rusted .22 rifle. The bones were still clothed in a very soiled running suit. Decomposition of the flesh had thoroughly soaked the running suit and left it in a dry, hard, crumpled mass. There was a .22-caliber gunshot wound in the forehead of the skull.

The police brought me the body and the clothing and asked me for an analysis.

It was a small skeleton, a very *gracile* individual. I briefly examined the running suit and put it aside and turned to the bones. After a while I phoned the medical examiner's office and said: "I believe the individual is a male, probably from Asia and in his late twenties and of short stature." They thanked me and said they would check the missing persons reports.

A few days later they called back and said: "We've got some missing Asiatic females but no males."

I said I'd take another look at the skeleton. I called back and said that the pelvis showed some female characteristics, but overall I thought it was a male. They pleaded with me: "Can't you tell us anything more?"

So I went back and looked at the skeleton a third time. I pried open the hardened mass of the running suit and found a pocket concealed on the inside of the trousers. I removed several objects and called the medical examiner's office. After all this work I felt a smug satisfaction in having solved the mystery by very obvious methods.

"I can't tell you his name," I said innocently, "but would his address and driver's license number help you at all?"

Among the objects in the clotted-together pocket was a disintegrating driver's license that identified the owner as a twenty-eight-year-old male from the Philippines, who had been arrested a couple of years before for attacks on male children. He had escaped from custody during transport, hitched a ride in a pickup truck and leaped out of the truck with a .22 rifle stolen from a rack on the rear window. After that, he had vanished. Desperate, a fugitive, he had apparently decided to kill himself using the stolen rifle.

On February 17, 1818, a large tomb was found on the grounds of Dunfermline Abbey in Scotland. Sandstone slabs concealed a shallow vault, barely eighteen inches deep. Fragments of oak and nails and tatters of gold cloth were found around the form of a tall man, encased in lead. Immediately speculation arose that this was the long-lost grave of King Robert the Bruce, a hero of the Scottish wars of independence, the man who, according to legend, learned patience from a spider spinning its web at his cell window, the man who forced the English to relinquish their claim on Scotland in 1328 with the Treaty of Northampton. Yet King Robert's death had always remained a mystery. He died only a year after this personal triumph, shut away from the world, apparently in the grip of a mysterious wasting disease. He breathed his last, aged fifty-five, on June 7, 1329, and was buried in Dunfermline Abbey, his heart enshrined separately at Melrose Abbey.

The rediscovered grave was hastily closed up again and remained locked and barred until it was officially reopened on November 5, 1819. A large crowd of notables and scientists were on hand to witness the event. The lead was peeled back from the limbs and sawed away from the skull of the skeleton, which belonged to a man who in life had stood about five feet eleven inches tall. The breastbone was split, as if the heart had been forcibly removed after death. The teeth of the lower jaw survived, but the upper incisors were missing from the maxilla, or upper jaw, and the maxilla itself looked curiously eroded and worn away. The body was examined and an exact cast was made of the skull, which still reposes in the Anatomical Museum of the Medical School of the University of Edinburgh. A copy of the cast is kept in Dunfermline Abbey, and another in the Museum of the Royal College of Surgeons of England in London. The skeleton was then reburied with great pomp and ceremony, and a copy of John Barbour's 1375 epic poem on the life of Robert, *The Brus,* was interred with the bones. For the skeleton almost certainly belonged to the greatest of Scotland's kings, Robert the Bruce.

But the story did not end with the reburial. The unexpected revelation of the skull enabled investigators to settle once and for all a rumor about King Robert, put forward in 1327 by the French chronicler, Jean Le Bel. Le Bel said King Robert died of *la grosse maladie,* a medieval euphemism for leprosy. Today leprosy can be treated and arrested with such drugs as dapsone and rifamprin, but in the Middle Ages the visitation of the disease sentenced the sufferer to lifelong banishment and a lonely, lingering death. The disease germ, *Mycobacterium leprae,* hates heat and heads for the cooler areas of the body: the buttocks, the nose, the extremities of the limbs and, in males, the testicles. Here it multiplies and gnaws away at nerve endings and skin and cartilage tissue. As the nasal cartilage and the palate are destroyed, the patient's features undergo a kind of collapse, resulting in the classic "leonine" or lionlike face characteristic of leprosy. But because leprosy can mimic almost any skin disease, it is often very difficult to tell whether the "lepers" of the Bible or the Middle Ages really had the malady.

Enter Vilhelm Møller-Christensen. This Danish doctor, endowed with superhuman patience, had made a hobby of examining medieval skeletons in Denmark since the 1930s. In 1944, while working at Aebelholt Abbey in Denmark, he had unearthed the skeleton of a young woman whose bones were terribly deformed. He suspected leprosy, but to verify his thesis years of patient work were needed. He learned that medieval leper hospitals were usually dedicated to St. George (known as St. Jørgen in Danish), and that there had been thirty-one such hospitals in medieval Denmark. On the property of a farm near Naestved, known as St. Jørgen's Farm, long and patient digging revealed the most extensive medieval graveyard for leprosy victims ever discovered. Over a twenty-year period Møller-Christensen unearthed, cleaned and preserved more than 650 skeletons. Many had their upper incisors missing and their maxillae eroded, a deformity Møller-Christensen called *facies leprosa,* the "leprous face."

In 1968 the Danish doctor was finally able to examine the cast of the skull of King Robert. He needed only a few minutes' inspection to reach a conclusion. The ravages of *facies leprosa* were unmistakable. "The matter finally lay beyond dispute," wrote Michael Howell and Peter Ford in their engaging 1985 book, *The Ghost Disease.* "A

111

great man had been brought low by a terrible affliction. Robert the Bruce, King of Scots and a hero of his country, ended his days as a leper."

Perhaps the single most eloquent and affecting skeleton I have ever examined belonged to Joseph Merrick, the so-called "Elephant Man," whose story has reached a modern audience thanks to a popular play and motion picture.

For me, the Elephant Man is no artistic stage prop, nor a distant, historical footnote, but a deeply moving reality. I have carefully studied his bones, and these extraordinary relics made an indelible impression on me, I who have seen thousands of skeletons in every conceivable state of wholeness and decay.

I had two reasons for requesting to examine these remarkable remains. I wanted to look closely at Merrick's skeleton because it seemed to me that photographs and drawings of him in life showed distortions that did not particularly match the photographs of the skeleton. And since the skeleton and the body cast of Joseph Merrick were prepared immediately after his death and are both kept at the Royal London College of Medicine Museum, it was possible to use modern superimposition techniques to overlay one image upon another, the external body cast and the inner bones, matching them up. After an examination that lasted several days, we discovered that, to a surprising extent, Merrick's deformities belonged to his skin, not to his skeleton.

But there was another reason I felt it important to do this project. The museum's curators told me that at that time, in 1988 the American pop star Michael Jackson had made a startling offer to *buy* the Elephant Man's skeleton for a million dollars. The museum quite properly rejected his offer, but as soon as word of it got out, long-lost Merrick relatives came scampering out of the woodwork, eager to "rescue" the skeleton from the museum's collection. One may speculate as to their motives. I felt that, in the face of such demands to release this unique, famous and quite irreplaceable skeleton, it would be helpful to demonstrate that the bones of the Elephant Man could still contribute something to science. Human remains should not remain idle in museum collections. Medical museums are not attics in which to store things merely for curiosity's sake. Their contents should serve some ongoing scientific purpose. If the remains of Joseph Merrick were to stay in the collection, it was necessary to prove they belonged there. I hoped I was helping to "hold the fort," together with the museum's curators, against people who wished to traffic with Merrick's bones.

Nor was this a makework project. The diagnosis of the genetic disorder that Joseph Merrick suffered from has lately been called into question. Dr. Frederick Treves, who discovered the Elephant Man and wrote the original monograph on him, diagnosed Merrick as suffering from multiple neurofibromatosis. But recent articles have suggested that it might be Proteus syndrome, a newly discovered and rather obscure disorder.

Not being a pathologist myself, I didn't want to jump into that controversy, but I did want to make sure that the evidence of the skeleton and body cast was thoroughly used and would remain available to those pathologists interested in the question.

The Royal London College of Medicine Museum is a fascinating old building. Pacing the corridors of its upper floors, one feels the atmosphere of Victorian medical schools. I was there at Christmastide, 1988, and the building was like an icebox inside. I would come away from the hospital in the gloomy evenings, my breath fuming in damp dark, yet breathing the air of Charles Dickens, partaking of the spirit of some of the characters from *A Christmas Carol* or *The Old Curiosity Shop*. London is my favorite city, a veritable time machine, allowing you to slip back easily into bygone epochs simply by turning a corner, stepping into a narrow alley or shadowy byway.

Besides Merrick's bones, the hospital has a rich and macabre collection of oddities, including evidence of the famous 1911 "Siege of Sidney Street," in which police battled a gang of anarchists. There is a specimen in a jar—a bit of tissue with a bullet wound in it—taken from the body of one of the police constables killed by the anarchists.

To reach the floor where Merrick's skeleton was laid out for me, I climbed two flights of a back stairway. Just before the stairs, the walls were hung with the names and photographs of past medical staff members. There I saw honored Francis Camps, the famous forensic pathologist; Watson Jones, one of the premier orthopedic surgeons of his time; and Grafton Elliot Smith, whose magnificent study of Egyptian mummies remains one of the best ever done.

The Merrick skeleton normally resides in a large room in the museum. But for my examination it was moved to a small workroom, which contained among other things a large tank of tropical fish and a window looking down at the narrow street alongside the hospital. This view must have been very similar to the one once glimpsed by Joseph Merrick himself, for he spent his last years in two rooms of this hospital. The room we finally entered had an old-fashioned warded lock with a single plate coming down at the end, with a keyhole-shaped keyhole, which opened to a large old-fashioned heavy iron key.

There, facing us on a low platform, stood the famous skeleton.

I was surprised to see how small it was. Merrick had been a short man in life, and his stature had been shortened further by scoliosis, or curvature of the spine. I was also struck immediately by the great differences between the left and right sides of the skeleton. The bony defects were not at all symmetrical. Merrick's infirmity had invaded his right side utterly but spared parts of his left. The right side of his skeleton showed vastly greater enlargement and bony growth, while the left side was mostly lacking these defects. Even in the skull, the right side of the braincase displayed massive nodules of bone; but the left side was smooth and unaltered, except by the small rectangular window through which Merrick's brain had been removed during the postmortem preparation. This little window was closed with metal latches.

I measured the body cast, then the skull, from various directions. I prepared numerous video and photographic images, so that we could actually decide where his flesh met his bone, the exact thickness of Merrick's skin tissue. Thus we were able to establish exactly

114

how much of the abnormal growth was the result of soft-tissue tumors and how much was owed to bone changes. As I have said, we found that most of the changes in Merrick's head were due to soft-tissue abnormalities and not skeletal deformities.

Gradually, however, the cold light of science yielded to a host of human emotions. By passing my hand, very lightly, close to the surface of the massive body cast of Merrick's features, made after his death, I experienced a ghostly sensation: I could actually feel Merrick's hairs, stuck in the plaster after all these years, yanked out of his dead body when the plaster was removed after his death on April 11, 1890. These hairs may one day furnish absolute proof, by means of the DNA they still contain, of the exact nature of Merrick's malady. There may soon come a day when geneticists will be able to determine with certainty the genetic basis of Joseph Merrick's profound infirmity. Ironically the bones themselves are probably devoid of DNA; they were boiled after Merrick's death, prior to being mounted.

Other parts of his body were also preserved, including large areas of his skin with the major soft-tissue growths represented. Unfortunately the museum lies near the London Docks, a section of the city heavily bombed during World War II. During the Blitz, the alcohol in those old specimen jars evaporated and the skin specimens dried out and were lost. They would have been an ideal source of DNA.

Another small oddity: Dr. Frederick Treves, the famous surgeon who discovered and cared for Merrick, changed the Elephant Man's name to "*John* Merrick." No one knows why, and the error has crept into all the literature about Merrick, even the Blue Guide to London. But if one examines Treves's original notes, as I did, one sees that the doctor mysteriously scratched out the word "Joseph" and wrote "John." Merrick's birth certificate is also at the museum, and on this document he is clearly identified as Joseph.

This renowned and unique skeleton makes an almost physical impact upon your eye and heart. Perhaps it's because we have read so much about the man who owned it, and we possess such poignant descriptions of Joseph Merrick, his sad life as a circus freak, his remarkable rescue from misery at the hands of Dr. Treves, and his ennobling struggle to realize his human potential. For my part, I can only declare that this skeleton, perhaps more than any other I have ever beheld, *talks* to you in very simple, powerful, human terms. It transfers emotions to you in a physical sense, with a directness and immediacy unequaled by any other skeleton I have ever seen. As I looked at Merrick's hips—that oversized right hip, side by side with the undersized left hip—I seemed to behold poor Merrick himself, limping along with his slowly tapping cane; his outsize cap perched atop the great, swaying hood that curtained off his enormous head from mocking eyes; his shabby, concealing, ragged cloak: Merrick the man, as he was in life, making his way haltingly through the dark streets of Whitechapel at night, burdened with his terrible body. This image, I say, came to me with the vivid force of a vision, and it remains a haunting personal memory. As I beheld his hands, his delicate and almost perfectly formed left hand, and the huge, club-like right hand, I could see the two halves of Joseph Merrick, soul and body: the delicate, intelligent person caged within, who impressed all who came in contact with him with his essential humanity, his gentleness, patience and joy—and the dreadful, gnarled, outward facade of swollen bone and tissue run riot, which acted as a prison house to his spirit and made of him, to ignorant eyes, a monster.

Both these truths were written unmistakably in that extraordinary skeleton, and reconfirmed my faith in the veracity and expressiveness of the human frame. Stretched to its uttermost, deformed beyond deformity, bone never lisps, stutters or falls dumb. It proclaims its truths the more loudly, the more it is taxed and twisted by unnatural nature and misfortune. Patient and silent while we live, our skeletons shout to heaven and posterity after we die.

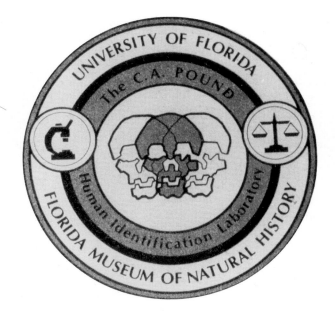

The logo of the
C. A. Pound Human
Identification Laboratory.

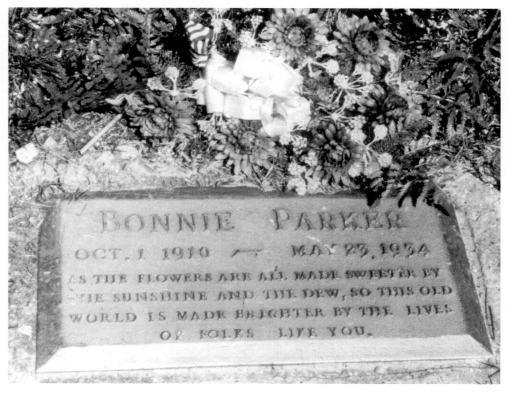

The tombstone of outlaw Bonnie Parker. Every criminal was likely loved
by someone in life.

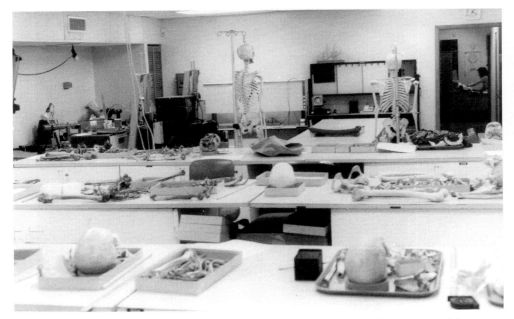

"These rough notes, and our dead bodies . . ." The science of forensic anthropology consists of listening to the whispers of the dead.

The C. A. Pound Human Identification Laboratory, showing "odor hoods." Inside these ventilated plastic bubbles skeletal remains are boiled clean of flesh and prepared for examination.

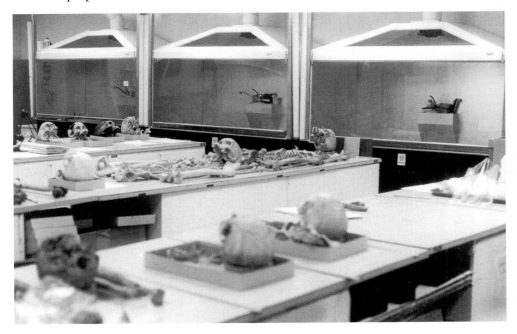

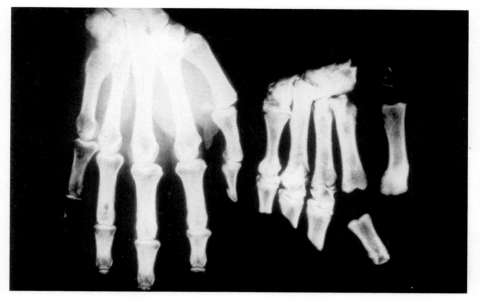

Nature's trickery: radiographs of human hand (left) and bear paw (right).

Male and female pelvises.
Note that the female specimen (below) has a greater
pelvic breadth and wider
subpubic angle. Such dis-
tinctions are aids in what we
call "sexing the skeleton."

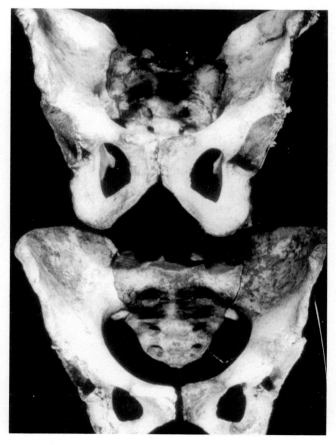

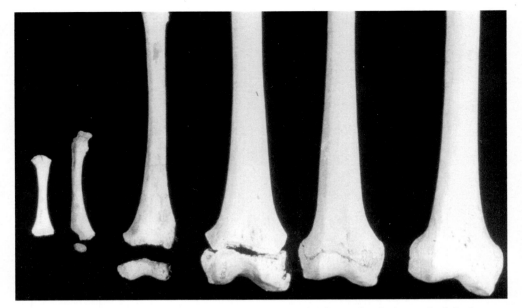

Human thighbones (femurs) as they progress through life. At birth the end of the bone at the knee is a separate element, or epiphysis. The epiphysis gets larger and changes its shape as growth progresses, beginning to unite with the rest of the femur. The groove, or scar, shows a femur that has recently united, signaling the end of growth. The groove disappears in an adult femur, and one might never guess the single bone had originally been several parts.

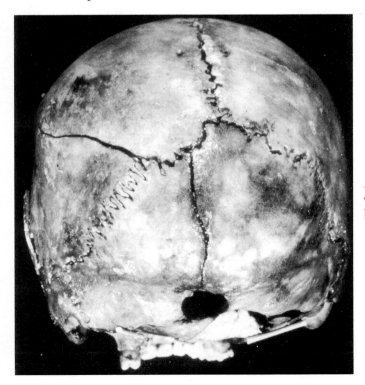

A .410 shotgun entrance wound at the base of the back of the skull.

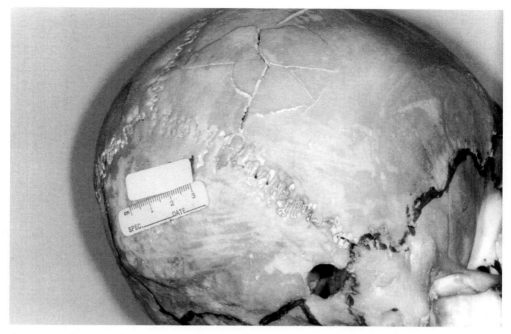

An incomplete gunshot exit wound. Note fractures near top of cranium. The round entrance wound from a second bullet shows no external beveling of the bone surface.

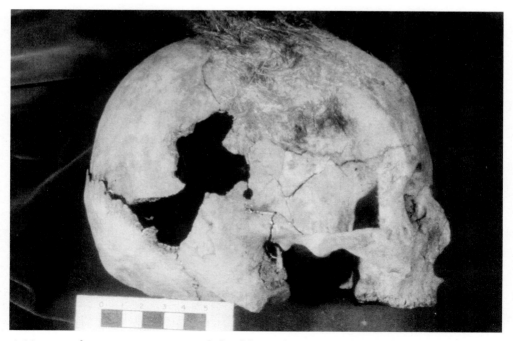

A 12 gauge shotgun entrance wound, fired from about ten feet away from the victim.

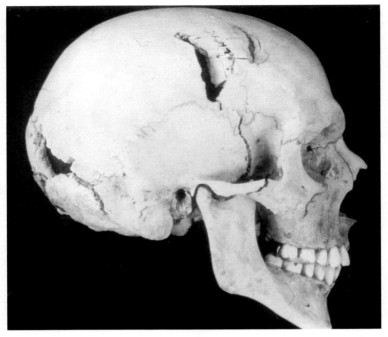

Skull showing multiple fractures from a tool.

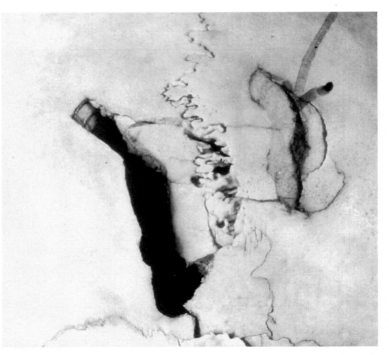

Which injury came first? This closeup photograph shows the injury on the left occurred before that on the right because a fracture (see arrow) from the left injury crosses the injury on the right. Therefore the blow on the left fell first.

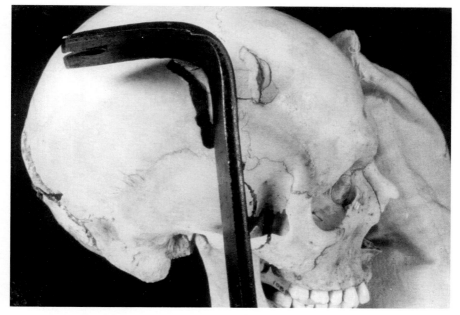

An apparent mismatch. When the tool is placed next to the wounds, it is not consistent. It has a right-angle bend. Such a tool would have cut smoothly into thin bone. Note that the top of the tool is ground down (dressed) while the shaft of the tool remains rounded.

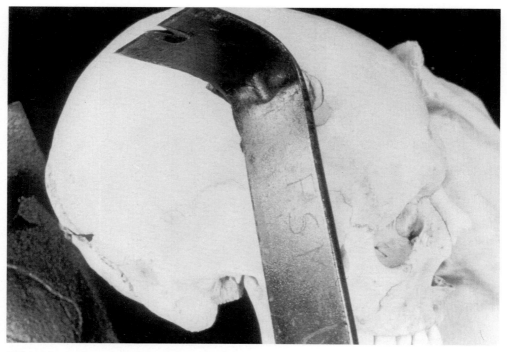

When the tool is rotated, however, the effective angle is now greater than 90 degrees. The tool would now crush the bone, causing the sloping surfaces seen in the wound.

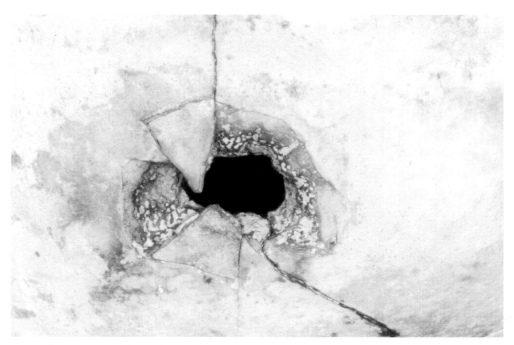

A gunshot exit wound, producing outer beveling of bone surfaces.

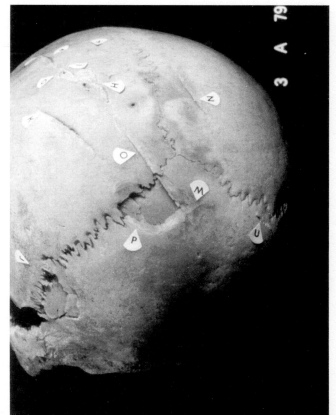

Multiple wounds from a
meat cleaver.

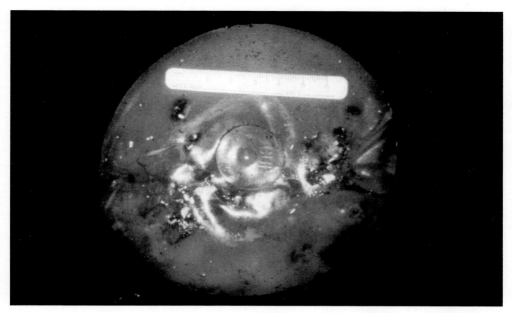

The size and manufacturer's trademark can be seen near the center of a silicone breast augmentation implant. One of my students once mistook this implant for a jellyfish.

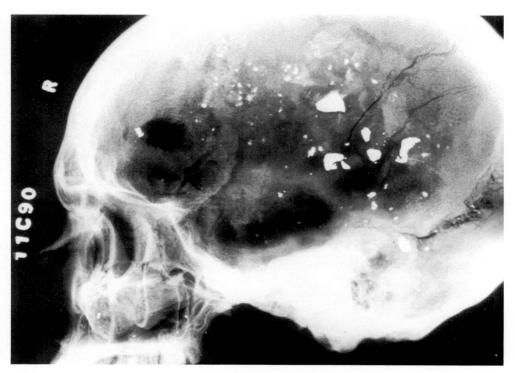

The many large white areas in this radiograph are scattered bullet fragments from multiple rounds of a .22 in the head.

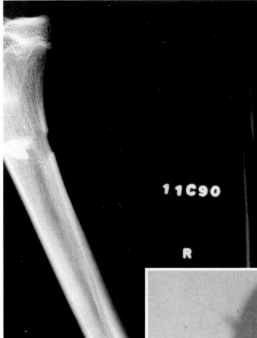

A .22 bullet can be seen embedded in a bone from the leg. The entrance wound in the back of the bone suggests that the victim may have been running from the assailant when he was shot.

The bullet tracks of five .22-caliber wounds to the head are indicated by the dowel pins.

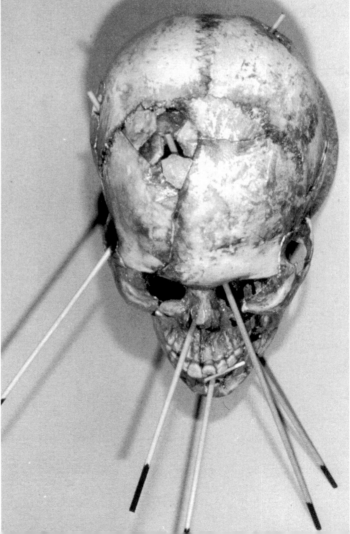

Vertebrae from the chest of an elderly man showing bony out-growths on the bodies and fusion of many vertebrae. In life, this man's movements would have been severely limited.

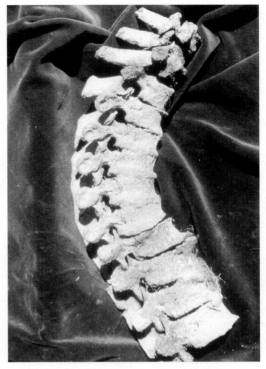

The La Belle drug murders. These three victims were bound and shotgunned and flung into a pit atop one another. The shoes of the murdered men appeared early on in the dig.

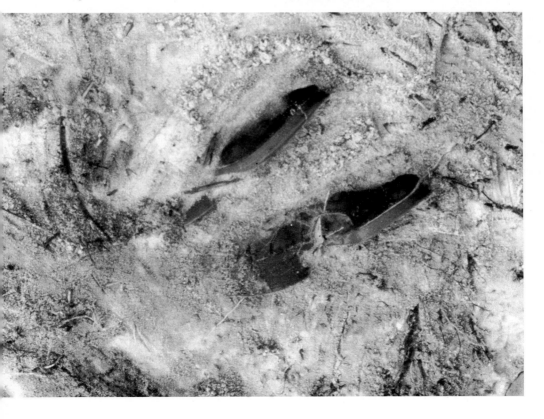

I am forced to lie beside the victims because of back pain. I found some relief from the heat and stench by drinking a Dr Pepper. *(Photo courtesy of Wallace M. Graves, Jr., M.D.)*

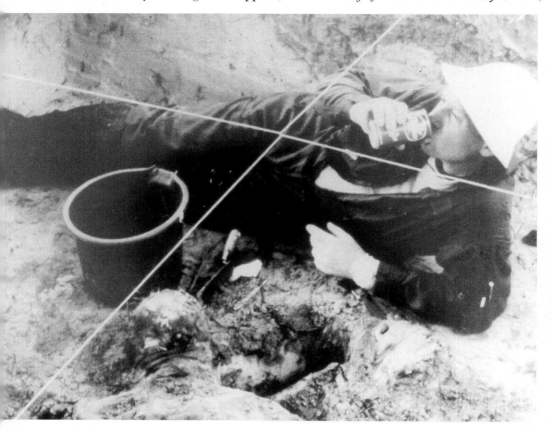

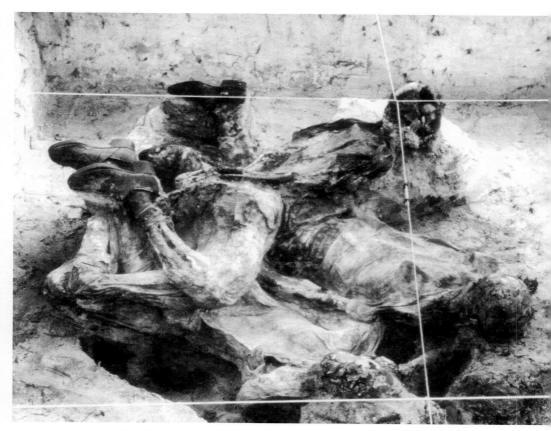

The three excavated bodies in the La Belle murder pit.

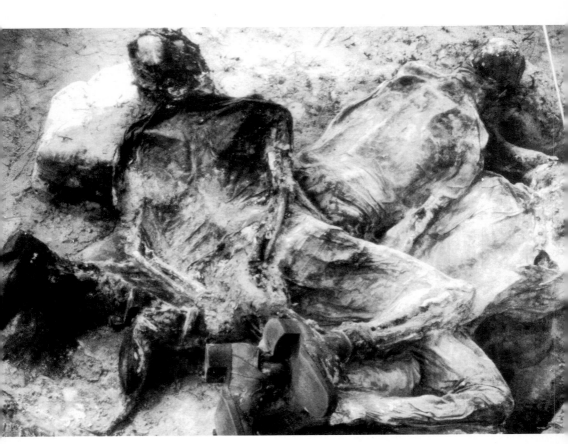

Another view of the three victims at La Belle. Our excavation demonstrated that the victim buried deepest had been shot last.

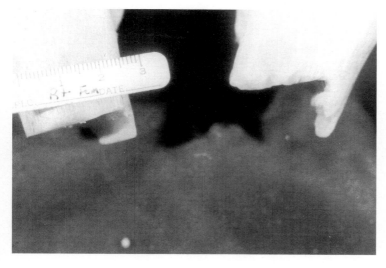

Femurs showing the typical pattern of chain-saw dismemberment.

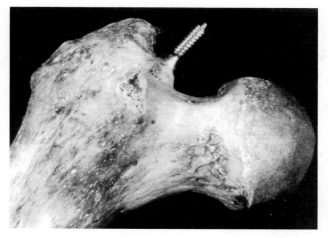

An orthopedic nail used to repair a fractured femur in life.

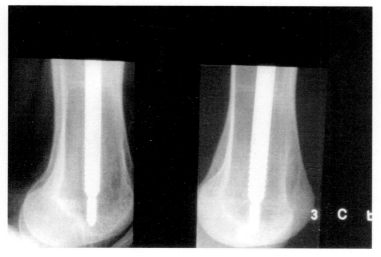

The bottom end of the same nail in life (left) and after death (right).

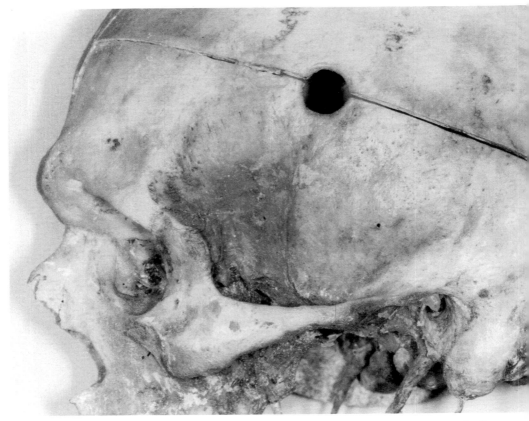

A healed hole in a skull (trepanning), drilled to relieve pressure after a head injury.

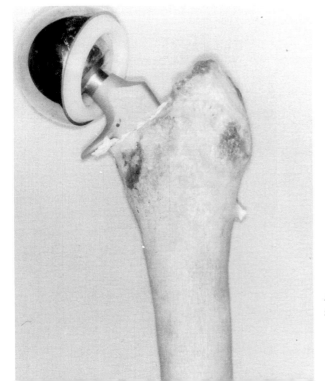

An artificial hip taken from a skeleton.

9

"A Sunless Place . . ."

Methought I saw
Life swiftly treading over endless space:
And, at her footprint, but a byegone pace,
The ocean-past, which, with increasing wave,
Swallowed her steps like a pursuing grave. . . .
So lay they garmented in torpid light,
Under the pall of a transparent night,
Like solemn apparitions lulled sublime
To everlasting rest,—and with them Time
Slept, as he sleeps upon the silent face
Of a dark dial in a sunless place.

—Thomas Hood, *The Sea of Death*

Hell is not a place, some theologians declare, but a state of being. Evil has no independent existence, St. Augustine wrote, but is merely the absence or negation of good.

Such subtleties lie beyond my competence. I am a scientist, not a clergyman. I do not know whence evil arises; but I have seen where it falls to earth, extinguishing life and disfiguring limb. I have examined carefully the aftermaths of evil, in that too late hour when it has already triumphed over the meek, the weak and the innocent. On my laboratory table I have read its atrocious language of wounds and outrages, the sight of which would wring the hardest heart.

And I have been present, too, at the autopsies of evildoers after they have been executed by law. I have seen the black scorch marks left by the electric chair on their shaved heads and legs; seen their brains and viscera laid bare by the knife and the Stryker saw, the tops of their heads popped off with a twist of the Virchow skull-breaker, a tool shaped like a large, shiny skate key with flanges on its bore. I have seen their organs lifted out one by one, set aside, weighed and photographed. Afterward, the autopsy room is thoroughly cleaned and disinfected with diluted bleach; but if you look closely, you can see that the bits of chalk used to scrawl the organ weights on the blackboard are maculated with old human blood.

On such occasions, we clearly do not expect demons to swarm gibbering from the opened braincase and flitter like black bats around the autopsy room. Nevertheless, it is impossible to regard a murderer's brain without an involuntary tingle of curiosity: what lay deep within the coralline gray whorls of this small, silenced kingdom? What happened along its intricate hallways, within the fine cerebral webwork of axons and dendrites, whose tiny, myriad sparkings are the physical basis of thought? Before it was shocked to death itself, what shocking poisons did this unique lump of flesh distill, to so subvert the mind of its owner and warp his will to evil?

I cannot say. Over the years my work has brought me into contact with abysses of evil: the most depraved murders, and the most unregenerate murderers. But even after long, enforced communion with the foulest recesses of human nature, I cannot trace this dark river to its source, nor can I suggest a way to dam or divert it. From what I have seen, the impulse to evil is something deep within an individual from his very earliest years, if not from birth. At the center of the labyrinth of certain human personalities there lurks a Minotaur that feeds on human flesh, and we have not yet found the thread to help us map this maze and slay the beast.

The instruments of murder are as manifold as the unlimited

human imagination. Apart from the obvious—shotguns, rifles, pistols, knives, hatchets and axes—I have seen meat cleavers, machetes, ice picks, bayonets, hammers, wrenches, screwdrivers, crowbars, pry bars, two-by-fours, tree limbs, jack handles (which are not "tire irons"; nobody carries tire irons anymore), building blocks, crutches, artificial legs, brass bedposts, pipes, bricks, belts, neckties, pantyhose, ropes, bootlaces, towels and chains—all these things and more, used by human beings to dispatch their fellow human beings into eternity. I have never seen a butler use a candelabrum. I have never seen anyone use a candelabrum! Such recherché elegance is apparently confined to England. I did see a pair of sneakers used to kill a woman, and they left distinctive tread marks where the murderer stepped on her throat and crushed the life from her. I have not seen an icicle used to stab someone, though it is said to be the perfect weapon, because it melts afterward. But I do know of a case in which a man was bludgeoned to death with a frozen ham.

Murderers generally do not enjoy heavy lifting—though of course they end up doing quite a bit of it after the fact, when it is necessary to dispose of the body—so the weapons they use tend to be light and maneuverable. You would be surprised how frequently glass bottles are used to beat people to death. Unlike the "candy-glass" props used in the movies, real glass bottles stand up very well to blows. Long-necked beer bottles, along with the heavy old Coca-Cola and Pepsi bottles, make formidable weapons, powerful enough to leave a dent in a wooden two-by-four without breaking. I recall one case in which a woman was beaten to death with a Pepsi bottle, and the distinctive spiral fluting of the bottle was still visible on the broken margins of her skull. The proverbial "lead pipe" is a thing of the past, as a murder weapon. Lead is no longer used to make pipes.

Whoever wishes to plumb the depths of man's inhumanity to man need only scan the textbook, the *Medico-legal Investigation of Death*, edited by two pathologists, Werner U. Spitz and Russell S. Fisher, one of the standard texts in our field. It is a 623-page tome filled with photographs that will sear the eyeballs of the uninitiated, though it holds no terrors for me and my colleagues.

In it are shown men, women and children in every stage of death and decay. Every refinement of murder and torture, every bizarre accident of fate and fortune, is laid out within these pages in dispassionate detail. Here are bodies shot, stabbed, hanged, bludgeoned, poisoned, mangled, decapitated, dismembered, flayed, drowned, strangled, stretched, crushed, burned, dried, mummified and plank-stiff with rigor mortis. Here are bodies that have been gnawed by dogs and rats, fish and alligators, beetles and roaches; bodies that are corrupt and frothing with fly eggs and maggots. And here, too, are bodies preserved with wondrous purity and freshness, enfolded soon after death in a bright crystalline coverlet of snow and ice, cradled by cold and seemingly immortal in their mortality.

But in many ways the most dreadful chapter in this Black Museum is Chapter Eighteen, which deals with the investigation of wrongful deaths in childhood. Its frontispiece is the body of a newborn infant, stabbed to death many times. One of the collaborators on this chapter, Dr. James T. Weston, calls child murder and child torture "man's inhumanity to man in its most extreme form," and he notes that this darkest of deeds has been "rationalized by virtually every justification known to man, including religious beliefs and practices, discipline and education and, to a large degree, economic gain." Children are so defenseless and so innocent that these crimes seem particularly horrendous. "Whoso shall offend one of these little ones which believe in me, it were better for him that a millstone were hanged about his neck, and that he were drowned in the depths of the sea," warned Jesus Christ in Matthew 18:6. A millstone seems a very light punishment, in my eyes!

Some of the cases and photographs in this chapter can break your heart. There is the child who was choked to death by pepper, which its parents forced it to inhale for punishment. There is the child parboiled over half its body by immersion in hot water. There is the child whose frenulum, the stringy halter connecting the upper lip to the gum, is torn because he has been hit in the mouth so often (a lacerated frenulum is a common finding in physically abused children). There is the baby beaten to death by a drunken father because its crying interrupted a TV football game. There are the looped weals on the back and buttocks of a child beaten with an electrical extension cord—dozens and dozens of angry weals on a child's small back. There is a terrible photograph showing blackened necrosis of the fingertips of a child "sustained in an effort to protect himself when repeatedly beaten on the head."

I do not recite these horrors for low effect. I have two children myself, both girls, now grown, with sons and daughters of their own. I can feel keenly the pain a normal father feels in his imagination at the mere thought of such brutal injuries. It costs me an effort, in my professional capacity, to put aside the outrage any human being must experience when brought into contact with these depravities. Yet put it aside I must, if I am to reach clear and dispassionate conclusions in my investigations.

The more we know about these affairs, the more alert we will be to their telltale signs. I hope sincerely that a day will come when the brutal parent or adult will stay his or her hand, if only through fear of being found out; from the certain foreknowledge that the old excuses—"She fell"; "I turned my back for a minute, and it happened"; "He's always so clumsy . . ."—will no longer hold water, but instead lead to swift intervention, prosecution and stern punishment.

I have had several cases involving young children and they have always remained vivid in my memory. One of the most disturbing of these involved the remains of a five-year-old girl which were brought to me for analysis. They were found in a cloth bag that had been thrown into a pond. Her mother and her mother's boyfriend were accused of murder. There was evidence that they punished the child by forcing her to stand in the corner of the bedroom for approximately ten days without food or water or other fluids. She was not allowed to lie down and, whenever she collapsed, she was forced to stand up again. In a diabolical refinement of cruelty, a note was sent to her school informing her teacher that her medications required that she receive no food or water during the day. The teacher, knowing no better, complied with the strange request, becoming an un-witting accomplice in the poor child's torments. Fortunately, she kept the note, and this telltale piece of paper was later used as evidence in the investigation of the little girl's murder.

For murdered she had been. An indictment had been secured which charged that the girl had died of a penetrating wound to the skull. My part of this terrible case lay in the interpretation of injuries and, after a careful examination of the remains, I decided that the death-by-head-injury scenario was false. The hole in the little girl's skull was natural. A small bone had simply fallen away from the decomposing skull, under water.

After I discussed my findings with the medical examiner, he returned to the district attorney and indicated to him the true cause of death: starvation compounded with possible blunt trauma caused by beatings on the abdomen. A new indictment was obtained, one that excluded the penetrating injuries. At the trial it came out that the little girl was forced to eat soap and recite the alphabet end-lessly. She was whipped mercilessly with a belt whenever she wet her pants. She was forbidden to sleep, but instead had to stand nightlong in a half-packed suitcase. The mother's boyfriend, a sadis-tic lout named Don MacDougall, was the child's chief tormentor. The mother herself plea-bargained with the district attorney in re-turn for a fifteen-year sentence. She has served her time, with time off for good behavior, and is already free. MacDougall was tried in early 1983 and was sent to prison. He was due to be released from the Madison County Correctional Institute in North Florida on New Year's Eve 1992. Under the old penal regulations, MacDougall had managed to shorten his sentence by a certain number of days, for good behavior behind bars. But when it was learned he was to be let loose, there was such an outcry from the community that the Florida attorney general, Bob Butterworth, intervened personally and re-scinded the early release date in MacDougall's case. As of this writ-ing, he is still behind bars, and as one who has seen the pitiable remains of his victim, I cannot feel sorry for him.

———

Sometimes it takes a long time to conclude a case. In 1983 a medical examiner from Naples, Florida, sent me the skull of another five-year-old girl. He wanted to know what kind of weapon had damaged the skull. As I examined the skull carefully, I found that something had struck the little girl in the center of the forehead and crushed her fragile bones through the inner halves of both eyes, then passed through her frontal bone, producing a defect that extended from the base of her nose sloping upward and backward almost to the center of the top of her head. It was a terrible injury, caused by terrific force. It must have killed her instantly.

After taking some measurements and looking at sharp angles formed by the crushed bone, I reported that the weapon had a flat surface, two sharp angles and parallel sides. It appeared as if she had been struck by the narrow edge of a two-by-four piece of lumber, or something very similar in shape and dimensions. That was all I could determine.

Years passed. Then, in 1992, almost ten years after her death, an investigator told me he had interviewed a pedophile already in prison, who had admitted that he had killed the girl. We had to exhume the rest of her body from the cemetery to gather additional evidence, but the confession of the murderer agreed very closely with my original findings. He told police he had used, not a two-by-four, but a piece of building block about an inch and a half thick. Its sharp angles and straight, parallel sides matched the injury to the little girl's skull exactly. Eventually he pleaded guilty to the crime and the case was finally closed. The little girl's skull, which had been separated from her body as evidence, has been finally buried with her.

Our first impressions are always the strongest. One case in particular has haunted me for years because of the powerful impression it made on me at the time, and because it was one of the first such cases I encountered. It involved the dismemberment of a young girl, just thirteen years old, and it occurred in 1978.

Her skull was found inside a paint can only a couple of weeks after the child herself disappeared from a school bus stop on the east coast of Florida. The skull was clean when it was found in the paint can and the paint can itself was rusty and had probably rusted before the death of the child. This detail was of some importance, as you will see. The rest of the child's body was never found.

My analysis disclosed that the cartilage covering the occipital condyle, the bone that supports the skull on the neck, had been cut on its forward surface and bent backward, while the cartilage was still fresh. Now when I first saw this skull, after the police brought it to me, this tab of cartilage had dried, blackened and hardened, but a microscopic analysis showed that the cuts had been made before this drying and hardening took place.

The conclusion was obvious and grisly: a knife had been used to remove the head from the bones of the neck immediately after death. Additional cuts were found in various places on the skull, some in places deep within it, places where even a knife used in the most ferocious assault could not reach. I concluded that a knife had been used to *deflesh* the remains after death.

There was a fracture of the upper jaw which probably resulted from a blow under the chin. So blunt trauma had taken place; the young girl had been hit hard, perhaps hard enough to kill her, almost certainly hard enough to knock her unconscious.

Rusty scratches parallel to one another were found on the top of the cranial vault. Now, since the police investigators had carefully cut the paint can apart and spread it open to remove the skull, we could surmise that these scratches occurred when the skull was forced through the rusty rim of the can by the murderer. That meant that there was no soft tissue on the skull when it was forced into the can. It must have been boiled, to have been rendered so clean in so short a length of time.

Bone during life is covered with a very tough fibrous material called periosteum. Pardon the illustration, but when you eat barbecued ribs, the tough fibrous material that makes the meat adhere to the ribs is the deceased pig's periosteum. In the case before me, I concluded that, even if shreds of periosteum had been left on the

124

skull when it went into that paint can, those rusty scratches could not have been made on the surface of the bone. Therefore all the periosteum had been carefully and thoroughly removed by the killer.

Gradually a terrible picture emerged. Abducted, beaten, murdered, decapitated, her skull scraped clean with a knife and then boiled and jammed into a rusty paint container—the little girl had met a cruel and terrible fate. Though her identity was established, and the time of her abduction was pinned down, no arrests were made.

Often in the years that followed I thought about that small, pathetic skull. Some years later I asked to see it again, hoping that with experience and hard-won expertise I might spot something I had missed in my first analysis—in vain. I had learned all I could learn from it. I was almost resigned to the fact that not all murders can be solved and that this little girl was among those innocents whose deaths go unavenged. The only bitter consolation in this case was that the girl's parents knew what happened, and that their daughter was dead beyond a doubt. So many cases of missing children are never resolved; and the parents remain in agonies of uncertainty for the rest of their lives, always clinging to the faint hope that the child may still be alive somewhere. In such cases the lives of the parents are often wrecked forever.

Then, in the early part of 1994, as this chapter was being written, a man was arrested in New England in connection with the murders of several twelve- and thirteen-year-old children. I learned that he lived in the same county as the decapitated thirteen-year-old whose skull I had examined so carefully. At the same time, another twelve-year-old girl was murdered in an adjoining county, in a case I had also investigated at the time. I have passed the case numbers on to investigators. I hope that a demonstrable link can be found. I hope that the law has caught up with a monster.

Sometimes we get confirmation of our findings from the murderer's own lips. In 1990 a man named Michael Durocher, who was on Death Row at the Florida State Prison in Starke for another crime, and who saw his appointment with the electric chair draw ever nearer, decided to get certain matters off his conscience.

Durocher told investigators where he had buried his girlfriend, Grace Reed, her five-year-old daughter, Candice, and his own six-month-old son, Joshua, all of whom he had murdered some ten years earlier. Durocher was under a death sentence for the 1986 shotgun slaying of a Jacksonville store clerk, whom he robbed of forty dollars and a car. He had also been convicted of fatally beating a roommate in Jacksonville in 1988, and received a life sentence for that crime.

Now, in 1990, following Durocher's directions, a team from the Florida Department of Law Enforcement (FDLE) located the bodies of the children, Candice and Joshua, as well as that of Grace Reed, in hidden graves in Green Cove Springs. Durocher admitted that he shot the mother and daughter with a shotgun, but when investigators asked how the baby died—this baby was his own son—he suddenly fell silent. Then, with a grim smile, he said cryptically: "That's for you to find out."

Indeed, forensic analysis clearly showed that the woman was shot in the back of the head with a shotgun and the jacket and bones of the little girl showed that a shotgun blast hit her in the back near her right armpit and tore through near her breastbone.

But the bones of baby Joshua had not a single mark on them. Clearly he was not killed with a shotgun. Was he stabbed? Smothered? Choked? Or had he been buried alive? "That's for you to find out," Durocher had said. I took him at his word and accepted the challenge. With infinite care, I bent my attention to the tiny, mostly skeletonized remains before me, which belonged to an infant murdered ten years earlier.

The ribs were not in good condition, but as far as I could see there were no nicks on them. They were clean. In cases of stabbing murders involving adults, the stabbing implement will not strike any bone about fifty percent of the time. In children, the probability is obviously much higher, because children's bones, especially their ribs, are much closer together. But in this case there was no sign of bone damage.

The baby was still dressed in overall rompers with a bib going up to straps across his shoulders. The legs opened on their inner seams so that his diapers could be changed. Under the bib of the overalls was a T-shirt with hearts and balloons on it and over the clothing of the upper body was a jacket with a hood. All the snaps on the rompers were closed. The straps at the top of the bib were fastened, the shirt was in place under the straps and bib. The top snap of the jacket was closed, but the lower two snaps were opened.

We photographed the clothing still in place and could see no perforation in the back, in the front, or anywhere. But then I discovered that, if I raised the lower corner of the unsnapped jacket and peeled it back, there was a perforation in the bib. When I examined the T-shirt beneath the bib, I found another perforation, with the same tilt of its axis, in the same location as the one in the bib. Under the microscope the synthetic threads could be seen to have a sharp, slanted cut at their ends.

I reported my conclusions to the prosecutor and the defense attorney: that in my opinion the child had been carefully stabbed to death, by a murderer who was fastidious enough to lift the corner of the baby's jacket, slip the knife in through the two layers of clothing underneath, and then coolly replace the jacket over the dying infant's fatal wound.

I was quite confident of my conclusions, but apparently the prosecutor was not. Later, however, Durocher broke down and pleaded guilty to first-degree murder in these three deaths and was given three more death sentences. After his conviction, the text of an interview he had had with a prison psychiatrist was made available to the court. The prosecutor telephoned me, excitement tingling in her voice, and told me that I had been right. Durocher had confessed to stabbing the baby in the left chest, underneath its jacket, just as I had said. I told the prosecutor I was not surprised, that I had been confident I was right all along, and that she ought to have trusted me more. Was I arrogant? I hope not.

Durocher went to the electric chair in the fall of 1993. At the end he behaved stoically, refusing to beg for clemency, or to pursue legal appeals, or even to seek a stay of execution. To Florida Governor Lawton Chiles he wrote forthrightly that he believed in capital punishment and added: "I respectfully request that justice now be served." It was. Michael Durocher is no longer among us. Unfortunately, neither are the five other people he senselessly murdered, including his own infant son.

Because of my connection with the case, I was invited to be present at Durocher's autopsy but had to decline, because I was to be in Hawaii that day, working with some Vietnam War remains. In Florida, executed criminals are not autopsied in prison. After being electrocuted and pronounced dead, they are loaded into a funeral coach and taken to the District 8 medical examiner's office in Gainesville.

When one is present at such autopsies, one's thoughts naturally revert to the question of capital punishment. I suppose I have an idealistic, humanistic admiration for countries like Great Britain that have abolished the death penalty altogether; but when I return to my work in the United States I conclude reluctantly that we Americans may not yet be sufficiently advanced to take that sublime step. I have seen cases—too many cases—of people who have served time for one murder killing again after being released. I have seen the bodies of prisoners murdered in jail by killers who are still serving time. I once saw the mutilated corpse of a prisoner who had been handcuffed, stabbed through the eyes and in other parts of his body, then thrown off a third-floor balcony inside the prison.

Capital punishment is a kind of "scorched earth policy," a last, desperate resort. We create a kind of sterile dead zone around a murderer and his deeds, a sort of "blasted heath" like that in Shakespeare's *Macbeth*, where nothing lives, except for evil fogs and ghostly warnings. The murderer is gone, his victims are gone, and all that remains is a frightful memory, together with the grim certainty that the dead man will never torture, taunt or kill again. The families of his victims, however, inherit lifelong grief, never to be consoled.

As for the various methods used to inflict capital punishment, I believe some of them are needlessly cruel. Hanging can be anything from a merciful narcosis, to an excruciating agony of strangulation, minutes long, to outright decapitation, if the condemned person falls too far. There is a classic article on hanging, published in 1913 in the British medical journal, *The Lancet.* Ideally, hanging dislocates the neck between the first and second cervical vertebrae, producing a fracture of the odontoid process of the second vertebra, which extends up into the arch of the first. This severs the spinal cord and prevents further respiratory function, as does the rope itself, which constricts the airways.

But it is almost certain that the brain survives conscious for some seconds, maybe even half a minute, after the drop. In some botched hangings, like that of Mary Surratt, who was alleged to have conspired to kill Abraham Lincoln, the body may twitch horribly for several minutes. This is how long it takes for the brain to exhaust the oxygen that was sent to it during the last instants of life. I know that many hangmen in their autobiographies have boasted of their skill, asserting that "the body never moved after the drop." This means nothing. With the spinal cord severed, the nervous system has been truncated, and no messages can be sent to the lower limbs. But the brain most likely still lives yet a little while longer, in agony, inside the "command module" of the separated skull.

Neither does the guillotine extinguish life in an instant. Grisly experiments involving signals sent by means of eye blinking have verified that brain activity continues for twenty to thirty seconds after death, in a guillotined head. Our brains continue to operate as long as they have oxygen, and when oxygen is lacking, they shut down. A guillotine merely cuts the windpipe and blood supply and nerve endings, but it takes a few seconds for the brain to feel the effects of the sudden deprivation of oxygen and blood. The condemned man, his heart beating wildly with fear, his lungs pumping furiously, is involuntarily prolonging his own agony, richly supplying his brain with blood and oxygen, which will enable it to retain consciousness for several more painful seconds than it would otherwise, after the knife falls. I imagine guillotining must be apocalyptically painful. There is certainly a huge shock, related to the terrific trauma of the vascular and nervous systems.

Nor is the gas chamber any more humane, in my opinion. Hydrogen cyanide gas doesn't have the instantaneous effect in all individuals that is commonly supposed. There are numerous descriptions of prolonged gasping in some executions. This particular form of execution is unique in that, unlike any other method of capital punishment, it involves the cooperation of the condemned man. He has to take the fatal breath on his own, usually at a sign from the warden or executioner. There have been instances of breath holding on the part of the condemned man, in a desperate attempt to prolong life by a few more seconds. The final, involuntary gasping makes gassing almost a participatory, voluntary act. There is something vaguely obscene about forcing someone to kill himself.

We in Florida carry out death sentences by electrocution, which is supposed to be painless and instantaneous. I hold no brief for electrocution, but I believe it may be the least cruel of all methods of capital punishment, save one. When I was a college student working at a mental hospital in Texas, I was often called upon to take care of psychiatric patients before and immediately after they were given electric shock treatments. This involves a relatively small, nonlethal amount of electricity being sent through the brain. Without exception, I saw them lose consciousness instantly and never complain afterward of any pain, upon reviving. Indeed, not a single one of them could even remember the jolt. Therefore I believe the tremendous charge of electricity sent into the human brain during electrocution must pretty well scramble the nervous system, making it impossible to sense any pain.

If it were up to me, I should prefer that capital punishment be carried out exclusively by lethal injection. Unfortunately those opposed to the death penalty—and I readily grant they are acting from pure and humane motives—have raised all sorts of legal obstacles in the way of this much-needed reform.

During the administration of a lethal injection, a cocktail of chemicals is injected into a vein of the condemned criminal. This cocktail paralyzes the respiratory functions, stops the heart by the action of potassium chloride and closes down the brain quietly and painlessly by means of barbiturates. There have been many cases of suicides involving similar barbiturates, which are used to put animals to sleep. In most of these cases, the needle is found still sticking in the arm of the dead victim and usually the plunger is not even fully depressed—it is that quick.

Obviously, the only painful aspect of lethal injections is the occasional difficulty of finding a vein. Getting the needle into the circulatory system of individuals who have been drug abusers for years can be next to impossible. Physicians, too, balk at administering this final, deadly viaticum, because it violates their Hippocratic oath to, "first, do no harm." Paramedics perform the task instead. These qualms are nothing new. If you recall, in Plato's *Phaedo,* a doctor does not administer the hemlock to Socrates. Instead, a prison attendant brings in the cup, gives a few instructions and leaves the cell. Socrates drinks down the lethal potion himself.

I suppose the most infamous man I ever saw autopsied was the serial killer, Ted Bundy, who was electrocuted on January 24, 1989, after many appeals, for murdering at least thirty-six young women. Bundy's body was brought to Gainesville under tight security and autopsied at the medical examiner's office. I remember there were a number of young men dressed up in green scrub suits, trying to get past the hospital security men by telling them they were doctors in their residencies there. They weren't, of course; they were journalists. None succeeded, though a photograph of Bundy's autopsied remains was later snapped, after the body had left the M.E.'s office, and published in a supermarket tabloid.

Several things surprised me about Bundy when I saw him for the first time in the flesh. First, he was a much larger man than I had imagined. Somehow, looking at photos of him during the trials, I had received the impression he was slight, of medium height. But he was a tall, powerfully built individual. He had put on weight in prison. He obviously had been exercising well. Another interesting detail was his tan. Bundy exhibited no prison pallor, and one of the personal effects taken from his cell after his execution was a bottle of suntan lotion, the kind that works even without the sun. I believe there was a cunning reason for this. Right up until the end, Bundy had been negotiating frantically with the authorities, offering to go out west with them and show them where he had disposed of the bodies of his victims, in return for a stay of execution. Bundy had already escaped from custody twice, and I believe he was hoping to do it a third time. Tanned and fit, he hoped in his heart of hearts to give the police the slip and blend in with the population outside prison. If so, he was deluded. He died here in Florida.

The third thing that surprised me was Bundy's age. You could see it in his face. He had aged extraordinarily. He looked a lot older than he did during his trial.

As with all electrocuted criminals, there was a halo-shaped burn on Bundy's scalp, and a burn on the side of one leg. When the cranial vault was opened, there was the usual large mass of congealed blood on top of the brain that is common in men who have perished under these dismal circumstances.

An enormous amount of investigation has gone into examining physical brain structure, in an attempt to determine how the brain of a genius might differ from the brain of a depraved criminal. We all remember the scene in the 1935 movie, *Frankenstein,* when the bumbling assistant breaks the jar containing the "normal brain" and takes instead the brain of a criminal to be fitted into Dr. Frankenstein's monster. There is a brilliant and evocative passage in Carl Sagan's 1974 book, *Broca's Brain,* in which Sagan examines the cerebrum of the renowned scientist, Paul Broca, as it floats in a jar of preservative fluid. Sagan wonders if memories of evenings on the Quai Voltaire and the Pont Royal, of dinners with Victor Hugo, of passionate debates with other scientists, were still contained within the dead neurons of the floating brain before him.

But, as so many behavioral scientists have demonstrated, the physical structure of the brain doesn't give us the answers to the problem of good and evil. In deficient brains, you get obvious anatomical changes, and in degenerative diseases of the brain, such as syphilis, you get microscopic and even gross changes. But in general appearance the brain of a genius, a madman, and an imbecile may show no differences at all. Size has no bearing on intelligence. Some of history's most remarkable individuals had brains far below average in size. The brains of males are on average larger than those of females, but this means nothing, as I am sure many women will attest. The brains of modern humans are, on an average, smaller than the brain of an average Neanderthal.

No. If evil is to be found in the brain, then it is probably there from the very earliest years of life, and involves something very basic in the individual's personality.

When it finally was removed and examined, Ted Bundy's brain looked like anyone else's.

10

Flames and Urns

The shades are no fable: death is not the end of all, and the pale ghost escapes the raked-over funeral pyre. . . . Cynthia appeared to me, seeming to bend over my couch's head. . . . Her hair, her eyes were the same as when she was borne to the grave: her raiment was charred against her side, and the fire had eaten away the beryl ring her finger wore. . . . Spirit and voice yet lived, but the thumb-bones rattled on her brittle hands. "False heart!" she cried. . . . "Now let others possess thee! Soon shalt thou be mine alone; with me shalt thou be, and I shall grind my bones against thine, commingled!"

—Propertius, *Elegies, IV, vii*

To behold a human body, soul-sped and committed to the flames, slowly being combusted within the retort of a crematorium is to witness a spectacle at once solemn and strikingly colorful.

This is the ultimate bonfire of the vanities, in which all that we wore in life is brightly, briskly swept away like dross, leaving only the durable, solid bones beneath. If the door of the oven be opened during cremation, one can peer in and see the devouring fire playing over the image of mortality, which lies statue-still and stoic beneath the nearly colorless jets of faint blue burning gas. The slow reduction of the body is a very eerie sight, and as the skeleton emerges the flames turn different colors, when various salts and chemicals within us are caught and volatilized. Warm yellows and oranges predominate, with here and there a twinkle of blue-green fire from burning copper, and a flicker of purple from potassium. Finally the bare bone peeps through, blackens as the carbon compounds in it are consumed, then fades from dark gray, to light gray, and at last to ashen white. The bones may twist and split, but usually the pelvis remains articulated, and the skull, though cracked open slightly by the fire, is nonetheless left largely intact and unexploded. Afterward its sightless eye hollows gaze darkly upward at the firebrick ceiling and the chimney flue, through which so much of what we were in life has fled in a plume of fine smoke.

I have been inside such an oven, called a "retort" by those who operate them, and have investigated closely the process of cremation and the remains that it leaves behind, in connection with a macabre lawsuit that I will come to later. The bricks were still warm from the sojourn of the last occupant, and I had to duck-walk along the V-shaped floor with its central groove, to avoid getting ash all over my trouser knees. I was careful to hold my elbows close, to safeguard a tweed jacket of which I am fond. Bits of calcined bone lay in the corners of the oven and I measured them carefully—I might be called upon to testify about them later. The burning-chamber was cramped, dark, odorless and devoid of soot, but it did not lack a certain powerful, dismal atmosphere. I had to use a flashlight to peer into its farthest recesses, and the beam of the lamp revealed the black, sunken holes hiding the gas nozzles, which normally provide all the light and warmth this gloomy recess ever receives. When I later telephoned Margaret and told her where I had been, she took it very well, all things considered. She knows, by now, that my work leads me into some odd nooks.

Flame does interesting things to bones, and part of my job is to examine human skeletal remains after they have been burned. You might think that the process of combustion would leave little to study, and that ashes would yield few secrets about the living being so fierily diminished after death. But you would be wrong. Flames can create, and urns can hold, some very lively stories.

Crematories are usually housed in separate buildings, standing apart from the funeral homes that operate them. Each one is different, and there is a wide range in the quality of the work they do and the pains they take in combusting and inurning human remains.

Most crematories have a sort of factory atmosphere about them. There are usually exposed air conditioning pipes overhead, a lot of metal duct work for the exhaust. Floors are usually of bare concrete. Machinery stands roundabout, used in processing the burned remains and putting them into proper containers. One very elaborate crematory I visited had a retort that was open at both ends, with doors at either extremity. One end opened onto a nicely furnished room finished with wood paneling and drapes and a chapel-like atmosphere, and the doors to the retort were faced with wood. The remains, encased in a casket, would be pushed in through these handsome portals, which would then be closed gently by the funeral director. The relatives, if they chose, could sit in this chapel-like room and wait for the cremation to be completed. The other set of doors opened onto the bare-floored processing room, where the ashes and bones would be winnowed through, crushed and poured into their final container by businesslike attendants. Most families elect not to stay, as the cremation process takes several hours.

There are considerable variations in the procedure and the equipment used, but what I am describing now is more or less typical of what happens during the process of cremation.

Bodies come to the crematorium, most often delivered by a funeral home or by a service that picks up the remains at the nursing home or hospital or wherever death took place. Some remains may come from a funeral ceremony and arrive fully clothed. The remains may still be wearing articles of jewelry. If the owner wore false teeth in life, these may still be in the mouth. Some corpses even wear eyeglasses, though obviously these are not of much use to them anymore.

Most crematories refuse to cremate remains enclosed in caskets, though a few still do. The most common container used is a large cardboard box, casket-sized, glued or stapled at the corners where it has been folded into shape from flat storage, with a shallow lid. The appearance is not unlike that of an oversized shoebox. Enclosed in such a container, the remains are rolled on a wheeled table like a hospital gurney up to the door of the retort, or cremation chamber. This retort is lined with firebrick and has a very rough interior. Usually the mortar is cracked and flaking from the heat of the flames. Retorts are constantly being repaired and remortared, because of the damage caused by heat within them. This rough, pitted surface has its drawbacks. Ash lodges on the surface of the bricks and cannot be entirely recovered. But metal cannot be used to line the retort, as heat causes it to corrode rapidly. Only firebrick will stand up to fire over time.

There is usually a groove running down the center of the floor, to trap the combusted remains and make them easier to recover. Natural gas is used to burn the remains and the temperature inside the retort reaches about 1,700 degrees Fahrenheit. A cheap crematory can be bought for a few thousand dollars, an elaborate one for hundreds of thousands. Some of the better ones are made in England and have modern conveniences such as timesets, where a computer monitors the temperature and other variables and controls the cooling.

After the gas jets are ignited, cremation takes varying periods of time, depending on the heat and the individual characteristics of the body. But usually several hours are necessary. Fat bodies tend to burn more quickly than thin, muscular ones, and I even know of a case in which a plump corpse burned so fiercely that the inside of the retort caught fire and was damaged.

When cremation is complete, all the organic components of the skeleton have been destroyed, first by charring, then later by complete combustion. They are burned away. The bones go from their natural color to black, as the organic material is carbonized. Then, as these organic compounds are combusted, the black fades to dark gray, to gray, to light gray and finally to white. When the bones are white, they are said to be calcined. They are now extremely brittle, but they still appear more or less normal. Bones may shrink under the action of fire, sometimes by as much as twenty-five percent. They may warp and twist and sometimes fragment into small little checkerboard designs, the way a safety-glass windshield shatters into little cubes. Very often the checking pattern does not completely penetrate the surface of the bone but only the outer aspects.

This shrinking and warpage and checking does not occur until the body is approaching the naked bone phase. If you look at bones under a microscope at various stages of their combustion, you will see interesting changes. Before burning, a section of bone will show all its interior structures clearly. After burning, the structures can still be seen, though canals will be closed off and shrunken. But in the mid-phase of burning, all is black and choked by carbon residue, and very little of the bone's structure can be observed.

There seems to be only a very loose correlation between the weight of the body and its overall mass on the one hand, and the volume of the recovered "cremains," as cremated remains are sometimes called for short, on the other. For most adults the cremains weigh about 2.2 to 8.8 pounds. It has nothing to do with what you weighed in life, but is probably related to what your bones weighed. A small, osteoporotic woman would produce a small amount of cremains but a large robust male with a heavy frame would produce more. The proportion of ash versus bone fragments in cremains is about fifty-fifty.

When the body comes out of the retort in this calcined condition, a trained osteologist can stand a few feet away, glance at the remains as they emerge, and tell the crematory employees the race, sex and approximate age of the deceased. In other words the identifying characteristics are still there. *Fire does not destroy them.* But what happens next is devastating.

The remains are removed from the retort, sometimes by sliding a tray out, but more often by the use of a large, hoelike scraper and a similarly shaped brush. The hoe rather reminds one of the croupier's rake used to haul in betting chips at a gaming table. The bones and ashes are swept into the groove in the center of the floor, then scraped down the groove into a waiting container. This metal container is then taken over to a place where a large magnet is set up. This magnet is similar in size and shape to an extra-heavy clothes iron. It is not an electromagnet, but it works almost like one. It has a key handle that, when turned, neutralizes or activates the polarity of powerful magnets inside the iron. Turn the key one way and the magnet attracts. Turn it the other and all the attracted bits of metal fall off instantly.

During this process the heavy magnetic iron is used to crush the fragile calcined bone, like a hammering pestle. At this time, any large debris is removed from the cremains, including such things as hip prostheses, orthopedic plates, bridgework, any hardware from cremation containers, cardiac pacemakers and the like—although pacemakers are not supposed to be cremated, because their batteries explode. Crematorium workers look carefully for the wire leads that betray the presence of a pacemaker in the chest, and if one is spotted, it will be removed before cremation. But the leads are small, and it is difficult to spot them every time. These fragments of nonferrous metals are separated out and usually thrown into a garbage can: they are not considered an integral part of the body, and they seldom find their way into the urn.

Silicone breast implants are a funeral director's nightmare, as they tend to pop open and melt messily all over the inside of the retort. Hence, no effort is spared to detect and remove them before the rest of the body is burned. If they are not subjected to fire, these bags of silicon are wonderfully indestructible and will long outlast their owners. I have found breast implants around scattered skeletons that have decomposed in the open. We had a case in central Florida in which we were examining a female skeleton and its personal effects. One of my female graduate students, who had led a sheltered life, was watching while I found and poked a breast augmentation implant. It jiggled like a jelly-filled bag. "I don't understand," the student said innocently. "What's a jellyfish doing this far inland?" It took her a long time to live that error down!

To return to the cremation process: the crudely sorted remains are next placed into a "processor," which is a euphemism for a grinder. The grinders work in various fashions, but the most common types grind the remains until the particle size is small enough to pass through holes in a curved sievelike plate at the base of the processor. This is called the screen. The holes are about five millimeters in diameter, a bit smaller than a kernel of corn.

The processing is now complete. The cremains, after passing through the perforated plate, now consist of ash and various particles up to the size of the openings in the screen. They now are poured into the urn or whatever temporary shipping container the family has arranged. Sometimes they exceed in volume the size of the chosen urn, and the family has to be asked if they want to buy a bigger urn. If they don't, it is the duty of the funeral director to tell them that the excess ashes will be disposed of according to law. In practice, they used to be dumped in a common pit near the crematory. Nowadays, they are usually sent to a cemetery, to be poured into a common grave set aside for this purpose.

One very important step needs to be mentioned: before the cremation, most crematories place a nonferrous metal plate or disk with an identifying number with the body. This plate is incised with a five- or six-digit number that is used one time, and one time only, to identify this particular set of remains. If the disk is made of aluminum, it has to be removed from the remains before burning, and put back in with the ashes. If it is made of brass, it can stay with the body in the retort, as brass melts at 1,810 degrees Fahrenheit. This tag is usually recovered when the retort is cleaned and the remains are swept out. It will then be separated out before the crushing phase and dropped into the urn with the processed cremains. The number is logged in the records of the funeral home. The purpose of this tag is obvious: to assure that a certain set of remains ends up in the proper urn. It is all rather reminiscent of the bracelets given to newborn babies at hospitals, to make sure they won't be mixed up. Newborn or newly burned, we often look very much alike.

Some crematories remove jewelry from the remains before cremation and then place the uncremated jewelry in the urn. Others go ahead and cremate jewelry with the remains, remove it during the examination for metal prior to grinding, and then place it in the urn with the ground remains. Most jewels, incidentally, stand up very well to fire, as they were formed originally deep within the earth at temperatures significantly higher than a gas flame. Artificial rubies, for example, can be crystallized synthetically by gem makers using an apparatus called a Verneuil furnace, but only at 2,000 degrees Centigrade. Synthetic diamonds can only be crystallized at a pressure of 200,000 atmospheres, at a temperature of 2,600 degrees Centigrade. Real gems are formed at even higher temperatures and pressures, and the burning jet of natural gas in the retort is powerless to dissolve them.

As for dental work, the porcelain crowns on teeth will slump, but not melt, in a crematorium retort; and dental gold and silver will not melt at all. Sterling silver begins to melt at 1,650 degrees Fahrenheit. Gold melts at about 1,945 degrees Fahrenheit. Dental gold has an even higher melting point because it is an alloy, not pure gold. Amalgam tooth fillings or dental restorations will not usually survive the flames. They aren't found afterward. A strange material called "cremation slag," consisting of small lumps of grayish shapeless material, is often found. This slag takes the form of little beads. When broken open they reveal hollow interiors that appear to be made of glass, like tiny geodes. There are various explanations for how this slag forms: cremated hair, sand producing melted silicates, or chemicals from the bones producing a silicate-like debris. But it is almost always present.

Standard procedure does not permit more than one individual to be cremated at the same time in the same retort. Obviously the families expect that the cremains they receive in the urn will be those of their loved one and no one else's.

But in actual practice it is very difficult in a firebrick-lined retort to clean it out perfectly of all traces of previous occupants. Most crematories are very responsible. They attempt to do a professional job and adhere to the ethics of their profession. Occasionally, however, things go astray. When that happens, or when someone perceives that it happened, lawsuits fly; and this is when I may be called on to step in and investigate.

The claims raised in these lawsuits are varied: that the wrong cremains have been returned to the family, that cremains ended up in an unauthorized location, such as on the freeway, that infants were cremated along with adults, or that some trespassing stranger is kibitzing in the same urn with Uncle Frank. Vast sums of money are at stake. These lawsuits commonly demand millions of dollars in damages, and this is when I become involved.

Were you asked to make sense of this pulverized mass of burned infinitesimals, this tiny heap of ashes and calcined bone flakes, you would probably despair. How is it possible to reach back through the fire, to map and recreate what the fire destroyed? I tell you it can be done. I have done it.

When we are presented with these cases and we have to determine whether there has indeed been a switch or some other mistake, we have to look for far different evidence than we would with a complete skeleton. As you can imagine, the crushing removes most of the evidence of race and sex. Age may occasionally still be seen by arthritic lipping or outgrowths along a fragment of a joint, or a vertebra, or by dental structures, but such bone survivals are rare in the urn and usually so tiny they are extremely difficult to read.

In the case of immature individuals, such as infants, fetuses or small children, the immature bones may be extremely distinctive. Sometimes a very precise age estimate is possible. I well recall one case of cremated fetal remains in which I was able to determine the age of the fetus within a couple of weeks with great confidence, because of a tiny bone that survived the flames intact.

In most cases, however, what is really important, what tells the tale, isn't the remains of the individual, but the baggage they had with them. If you reflect a little you will see what I mean. Most of us carry around a surprising load of extraneous, artificial baggage inside our bodies, mainly because of advances in medical and dental science. Surgical procedures leave all kinds of inner footprints. After surgery to remove a gall bladder or a kidney, after bypass surgery, after a mastectomy, the blood vessels are clamped off with small metal clips. Because these clips are supposed to remain behind in the body, they are made of tough, rare metals that will resist corrosion. They may be simple stainless steel of very high quality, or they may be extremely unusual metals such as tantalum. These little clips can be cross-checked against surgical records at the hospital where the surgery was performed, and against the purchasing records of the hospital. These tiny clips, which will survive the flames of the retort, elude the pestle magnet because they are nonferrous, and will often make their way into the urn. They can be spotted amid the ashes often by the naked eye, more often (and more accurately) by x-rays. We can then have nondestructive chemical tests performed to assay accurately their exact composition.

Dental devices can also be helpful in identifying a cremated individual. Even though dental crowns seldom end up in the urn, dental *posts,* made of stainless steel or titanium, which are used to affix artificial crowns onto small tooth stumps, can be extremely important. Not only do they vary considerably in chemical composition, in size and in shape (each brand looks very different), but they are often altered by grinding the ends when the dentist inserts them into the tooth. These altered tips can be compared with dental radiographs or dental x-rays and be identified absolutely individually. They will show up in dental x-rays before death, and again in x-rays taken of the cremated remains. They can be as unique as fingerprints, because the dentist has shaped them to fit a particular tooth.

We also sift the ashes for stainless steel sutures used during surgery—heart surgery involves splitting the breastbone and wiring it back together—as well as various metal catheter devices used around pacemakers, screws in bones and a multitude of other things. If dentures are still in the jaws of the mouth when cremation takes place, the greater portion of them will be destroyed, but porcelain teeth, complete with their little metal pins used to affix them to the dentures, will survive.

What else do we find in urns? Sometimes the staples from the cardboard cremation containers, although the pestle magnet usually catches these. There may be the occasional screw from a pair of eyeglasses. Fibers and hair may show up under microscopic analysis, but these are most likely contaminants introduced after the cremation. They do not belong to the deceased but to crematory attendants who handled or examined the remains after the burning.

The examination of cremains requires the patience of a Swiss watchmaker. You need a microscope, tweezers, x-ray machines and boxes with grids so you can locate any minute metal fragments defined by the x-rays. If you x-ray a box of cremains and then try to sift the ashes, searching for that tiny little fragment that showed up on the radiograph, it is like looking for the proverbial needle in the haystack. But if you superimpose a grid over the outpoured cremains, then take an x-ray and study the grid, you can quickly localize the object.

Everything has to be carefully documented: weights, volumes and so forth. A lot of photographs have to be taken, and this can be painstaking, jeweler's work involving ultra-closeups or microphotography. One is always amazed at what can be found, as well as what isn't found. Just imagine, in a set of cremains, finding an ossicle, the tiny bone from the inner ear of an infant, intact! It takes a very solid knowledge of bone anatomy and variation and often a very vivid reconstructive imagination to identify these minuscule fragments of bone and metal.

Who pays me to do this sort of work? Attorneys, usually. They may be attorneys for the plaintiffs (Uncle Frank's near and dear ones), or attorneys for the defense (the River Styx Funeral Home), but they have this in common: they are at daggers drawn, deeply involved in a lawsuit. The greatest problem we have in these cases probably isn't the condition of the cremains. It's that someone is trying to save money and do an investigation on the cheap. These examinations take time, and time is money when you hire an expert. Minutes turn into hours, days, weeks. It has been my experience that the attorneys for the plaintiffs attempt to limit the time of the examination by their experts. By doing so, they are being penny wise, pound foolish. The less time spent sifting the ashes, the less useful material will be found.

By contrast the experts working for the funeral home are usually given adequate time to document everything fully. It is very embarrassing if you, the expert, fail to find something because someone said: "You have to do this in six hours," while experts for the other side are given six days to look at the same set of cremains.

You would be amazed how high the passions run in these cases. What I am about to reveal must be couched in careful terms, even though the case in question has long since been settled. I can give no names. I cannot even disclose which state this case occurred in.

A certain woman, much beloved of her family, died after a long and painful fight with cancer. She had had surgery when the malignancy was first found and then more than a year later it was found that the cancer had metastasized. During her final illness she had received very good medical care, with frequent x-rays and scans. She was cremated in the city where she died, and her cremains were shipped to a large cemetery in a nearby state. There, a set of remains thought to be hers was transferred from the cardboard shipping container to an urn, which was placed in a niche in the cemetery columbarium, where they were to rest in perpetuity.

That evening, someone found the temporary shipping container, with her name on it, on a freeway. Inside were cremains.

The family was tracked down and the box returned to them. They were outraged. They immediately retained attorneys and filed a $10 million lawsuit against the cemetery. Defense attorneys hired by the insurance company representing the cemetery interviewed forensic scientists from all over the country, searching for someone to put together a team of experts. The field of forensic anthropology is not crowded. My name inevitably came up.

I remember flying there for the interview, which was conducted in a suite of an airport hotel. I was surrounded by a phalanx of eight or more attorneys, who questioned me closely about what I would do, what should be done, what shouldn't be done and so forth. A short time after, I was told that I had been selected to put together a team of experts, the choice of whom would be left to me. The team assembled included Clyde Snow, who had worked with the Mengele remains in Brazil; Doug Ubelaker from the Smithsonian; Lowell Levine, one of this country's foremost forensic dentists, who testified at the trial of serial killer Ted Bundy; Bob Kirschner, a deputy chief medical examiner from Chicago; and Dr. Robert Fitzpatrick, this country's top forensic radiologist. One of the country's foremost microscopy labs was retained to do all the microscopic and chemical analyses.

By this point in the lawsuit the plaintiffs had been offered a very handsome sum to settle out of court. They refused. So we were told this would have to go all the way to trial. Our examination left no stone unturned. We lavished hours and hours upon our examination of the cremains. As our expenses mounted, the insurance company howled to the cemetery operators: "We promised you a Cadillac defense! No one said anything about Rolls-Royces!"

The medical records on the deceased woman stacked up eighteen inches high. The x-rays numbered in the dozens. We also had good dental x-rays. One of the important factors centered on the surgical procedure performed on the woman; the surgeon had used vascular clips to close off blood vessels. In the radiographs made before her death, I could count at least twenty-nine of these clips. Her surgical record indicated that the surgeon had closed off the blood vessels using Hemaclips, a special brand. Hemaclips are tiny things, about a quarter of an inch long. Hospital purchasing records showed that the hospital was using Hemaclips made of tantalum, although Hemaclips are sometimes made of other materials as well.

From the cremains in the urn in the niche, we recovered intact or in halves the remains of at least eighteen Hemaclips. The other eleven had been pulverized in the cremation and grinding process and were scattered uniformly throughout the ashes and cremains. These little specks could nevertheless be spotted by x-rays and chemically analyzed. Every single sample of cremains in the niche showed tiny fragments of tantalum. The cremains found in the box abandoned on the freeway did not show these flecks and indeed had no tantalum fragments at all. So they could not have come from the woman whose name was on the box.

Furthermore, the urn in the niche yielded a dental post that had been used to attach an artificial crown. It had been altered on both ends by the dentist who inserted it. The alterations on the ends of the post were very distinctive because they were irregular. We had five views of this dental post in the deceased woman's x-rays. I was able to put the tooth we recovered from the cremains under one video camera, then put each computer-enhanced dental x-ray on the other video camera, and superimpose them. We came down, thread by thread, lining up every single screw thread on the post, to prove this tiny piece of metal was a unique specimen.

The results of our investigation were clear and unequivocal: we proved that the woman was in the urn, and in the niche, right where she was supposed to be. We proved that the cremains on the freeway weren't hers. After the very first member of our team gave a deposition under oath, the plaintiffs hastily settled out of court for what I gather was a vastly reduced sum. Settlements are always kept secret, so I don't know what the figure was, but the attorneys we were working for were glowing like sunbeams and seemed extravagantly grateful. I gather millions of dollars were saved.

Why, the reader may ask, if our case was so airtight, did the cemetery pay out even a nickel? I am no lawyer, but I imagine that the universal fear of the unpredictability of the American jury had something to do with it. A box containing cremains was found on the freeway, and the box had the woman's name on it. There was always the possibility that a jury might stubbornly conclude, in the face of all scientific evidence to the contrary, that the box, the name and the cremains were all the proof it needed to find for the plaintiff.

Soon afterward I was called in on another case, and when I quoted my rates the new attorneys were taken aback. They called the lawyers who knew about the freeway case. "Isn't he a bit steep?" they asked, as I later learned. And the lawyer from the freeway case said: "Pay it. He's worth whatever he asks." It is always gratifying to receive these little tokens of esteem. The money isn't unpleasant either.

Whose, then, were the remains in the box left on the freeway? They were never identified. We were able to demonstrate that they were the remains of several people scrambled together, and their volume was rather small. This led me to investigate the interior of a crematory retort chamber myself, as I have described above. Within, scattered in the corners and amid the crevices of the firebrick walls, was a small quantity of bone fragments and ashes left over from previous cremations.

I suspect, therefore, that a disgruntled employee from the crematorium surreptitiously gathered up these remnants, or others like them, and placed them in the box beside the freeway to cause grief to the funeral home. He certainly succeeded.

But in the end, the dreams of wealth or revenge, the loud legal cries of injury and outrage, the hypothetical millions of dollars demanded to redress this imagined wrong—all of these were reduced to ashes and smoke. All that remains today is a cool, silent urn in a distant columbarium.

11

Death in 10,000 Fragments

You will say that reality does not have the slightest obligation to be interesting. I reply that even if reality can escape the necessity of being interesting, hypotheses never can.

—Jorge Luis Borges, *Death and the Compass*

There is a stretch of I-75 about twenty miles north of Gainesville along which the great highway passes through a green and smiling landscape, all rolling fields and thick forests of pine and live oak. I can never travel this particular portion of the interstate without glancing over at a beautiful pasture that appears just south of the exit for High Springs, via County Road 236. This pasture has a solitary oak tree at its edge, then a dense stand of forest just to the west.

Sheltered under the eaves of this forest are the ruins of an old burned shack. Within those charred ruins, on January 28, 1985, were found the remains of two calcined human skeletons, so badly burned that they were almost reduced to powder. Next to one of the skeletons, welded shut by the fury of the fire that consumed the shack and its occupants, was an Ithaca Model 37 12-gauge shotgun whose stock had been completely reduced to ashes.

Today when anyone asks me which was the most difficult, the most fascinating and perplexing case I have ever encountered, I

149

answer without an instant's hesitation: the Meek-Jennings case. I have examined human remains, ancient and modern, famous and obscure, in Asia, Africa, Europe and South America, as well as all over the United States; but I had only to travel twenty miles from my front doorstep to encounter the most baffling and complex problem in forensic anthropology that has ever occupied my mind or challenged the resources of the C. A. Pound Human Identification Laboratory.

The Meek-Jennings case began with a hellish fire, and from the first moment it was possessed of a hellish complexity. That fire, and those skeletons, would occupy me and my students for the next year and a half. Many times during my inquiry a vital piece of evidence would dangle just out of reach, then, when grasped, would slip away or reverse its meaning. I had to unravel a set of remains that occupied only a few square feet, but whose tangled history reached from Alaska to Florida, across thousands of miles and a dozen years.

Everything about this case seemed to defy a simple solution. Things seemed to reduplicate themselves, multiply themselves, fragment themselves. At times we seemed to be gazing through a kaleidoscope instead of a magnifying glass.

At first we thought we were dealing with one fire; it turned out there were two. We imagined we were investigating two deaths; later we found out there were four. The deaths occurred in pairs, in two states, widely separated. There were two suicide notes, both of which looked fake. There were dozens and dozens of antemortem and postmortem x-rays to compare, some of them of very poor quality. Other x-rays, which would have solved the case in an instant, had been destroyed. A slip of memory on the part of a surgeon plunged us into difficulties that seemed insoluble. A crucial gold tooth inlay eluded us for months, while another tooth, found hundreds of miles away, cast the gravest doubt on our findings at that point. At various stages in our inquiry it seemed possible that the bones in the burned cabin were a macabre jest, deliberately put there to make fools of us, by a murderer gifted with almost superhuman cunning, a man so ruthless he would pull his own teeth and fling them into the flames, to throw us off the track.

"We are to go together so our ashes cannot be separated," boasted a suicide note found a few hundred feet from the fire. It was my task to prove this prophecy false.

Besides the skeletal remains of two individuals recovered from the fire scene, there were the burned remains of a dog, as well as the previously cremated ashes of a second dog, all mixed together. Before it burned, the old cabin had been an abandoned farmhouse, which meant that all sorts of flotsam and jetsam were found mixed among the ashes. Generations of animals, wild and tame, had died and left their bones for years and years beneath the house. Mixed in with the fragments was an accumulation of old bullets and cartridges, shoe eyelets, molten buttons and even an ancient Chinese coin.

If only I had been called in just two days sooner! The Alachua County Sheriff's Department thought I was out of the country, in Peru, and unreachable; in fact I had just returned to the United States the morning before the remains were discovered. I could easily have gone out to the burned shack and seen the remains *in situ*. Instead an investigator from the medical examiner's office carefully gathered up every single bone fragment she could find, placed them *in a single body bag* and carried them back to the medical examiner's laboratory. By the time they arrived they could not have been more jumbled if they had been run through a cement mixer.

When I finally opened the vinyl bag I was overwhelmed. Inside, totally commingled and crushed, were approximately ten thousand bone fragments, not counting bone that had been reduced to ash and particles of sand. In my entire career I have never seen such an impossible chaos of fragments, some broken by the fire to begin with, some broken even further by careless handling, all tumbled together in a hopeless, brittle welter of dust, cinders, calcined bone, stray teeth and sand. If the bones had simply been cut into ten thousand fragments it would have been easier. As matters stood, the remains had been jumbled twice, once by the fire and again by the evidence technician.

The deaths in High Springs, as it turned out, were linked with a particularly shocking and heinous double murder in New Hampshire that had occurred a few days earlier. Because of the notoriety of the New Hampshire victims there was a blaze of media attention. Newspapers in Massachusetts, New Hampshire and Florida followed the case closely. We here in Gainesville were being pressured by politicians and law enforcement officers from another state. The New Hampshire authorities made it plain they considered us incompetent rubes and hicks who, to hide our abysmal ignorance, were desperately trying to sweep the whole matter under the rug. In view of the fact that I spent a year and a half painstakingly reassembling those skeletons, I consider that a bit of an insult. Long after we submitted our conclusions and proof the New Hampshire state attorney pointedly disregarded them and kept the case open. He went on to become governor of the state, so I suppose you have to hand it to him: he knew how to strike a popular pose in the public eye.

But one of the most fascinating aspects of the Meek-Jennings case was the personality of the killer. To a degree unparalleled in most of my investigations, the mind of the murderer seemed to taunt us and puzzle us, beyond death, beyond the dissolving fires that destroyed the old cabin and its occupants. In this case, contrary to all common sense, love and death were mixed in equal proportions. The Meek-Jennings affair was one involving both passion and premeditation. Here were present the deepest, tenderest sentiments of romanticism, side by side with a depraved, homicidal rage. Here the fires of love were nearly all-consuming. They almost consumed the truth.

To this day I cannot fathom why nobody spotted the burning cabin when it caught fire. There was a Shell filling station on a hill at the County Road 236 exit of Interstate 75, hardly a mile and a half away. To me it seems incredible that no one saw the smoke or reported the blaze, unless it happened at dusk, or at night. But even then we are left with the astounding fact that the ruins of the cabin were only discovered on January 28, fully ten days after the fire.

When sheriff's deputies arrived at the scene everything had long since cooled. The masonry of the cabin fireplace was cold. All the galvanized tin roofing had collapsed on top of the ashes and the metal was cool to the touch. There was not a wisp of smoke. Trees upwind of the cabin were scarcely scorched at all, but those downwind, to the west, were blackened and charred fully forty feet up their trunks. This was dramatic proof of how hot the fire had been and suggests that there was a strong wind fanning the flames in a westerly direction.

When the investigators arrived, the collapsed corrugated metal sheets from the roof covered everything completely. Only when they began to remove the fallen roofing did they begin to see bones.

They found the bones side by side, with the burned sawed-off Ithaca 12-gauge shotgun at the feet of one set of remains. The shotgun had been welded shut by the fire, and its stock was wholly burned away. The position of the bone fragments seemed to indicate that two bodies, lying side by side, had been consumed by the flames. The second set of remains was closer to the door. Several Coleman gasoline cans were found in the ashes, missing their lids and showing no signs of having exploded. They must have been emptied out before the fire. The two sets of bones were scattered atop and beneath a wire mesh that seems to have been part of an old gate. Even though some bone fragments had fallen through the mesh, there were a few still on top of it, which demonstrated that the bodies must have been lying above this mesh when the fire started. Under the wire mesh there was something extraordinary: charcoal briquets, burned to ashes but still recognizable by their shape. Whoever had started the fire had placed a considerable quantity of charcoal beneath the bodies, to make sure they would be consumed as completely as possible.

Right away the investigators were confronted with an oddity: a single fragment of a female fibula—that is the long thin splint bone that backs up the main leg bone, the tibia—was found outside the cabin, near its entrance, some feet away from the rest of the female remains. This fragment was not as badly burned as the other remains, though it was broken off and charred at one end. How had it come to be outside the cabin, away from the other remains? We racked our brains over this and in the end could only theorize that it was flung there by the explosive force of the fire, before it had a chance to burn completely. The cabin was built of "fat lighter pine," which is full of resin and burns explosively. In such a fire, rafters would fall, sharp-edged sections of tin roof would come hurtling down, and fierce convection currents would be swirling from all directions. In fact the ashes of a fallen roof beam were found near the leg portions of the female remains. It's my belief that this bone was somehow broken during the fire and flipped free of the rest of the skeleton at some point. This fibula would later play a significant part in my investigation.

Several hundred feet away from these charred ruins a blue Fiat was parked in the middle of the field. In the trunk of the Fiat were found clothing and personal effects that identified their owners as Glyde Earl Meek, a forty-nine-year-old white male, and Page Jennings, a twenty-one-year-old white female. Meek's and Jennings's clothing was in the trunk of the car. There were his expensive-looking cowboy boots with their intricately tooled uppers and polished toes, his shirt, his blue jeans, a red windbreaker and his underpants, all folded up. Next to these garments, in a separate pile, were Page Jennings's white Reebok sneakers. One of the sneakers had a pair of sunglasses thrust into it and a bloodstain on the side. A baseball cap from the Stacks restaurant at the Gainesville downtown Holiday Inn, where Jennings worked as a waitress, was also in the trunk. Her flesh-colored bra and floral print panties were also neatly folded on top of the pile of her clothes, which included a white pullover sweatshirt and a green plaid shirt.

If the skeletons within the cabin were those of Meek and Jennings, then it seems likely they embraced the flames naked.

In the rear seat well of the blue Fiat were found tools, a jack

handle and a set of electrical connectors used to hot-wire the vehicle. Atop the back seat was an emergency first aid kit, a plastic coffee
cup and a towel. The cloth car seats were split open with wear and
tear.

On the front seat was a very long and very strangely worded
suicide note, written neatly in longhand on four sheets of yellow
legal paper, front and back. Counting front and back pages, the note
was actually eight pages long, an exceptionally long message as suicide notes go. The spelling was generally correct, except for the
words "separate," "supporting" and "appalling," which were spelled
"seperate," "suporting" and "apauling." The vocabulary showed an
above-average range, a good command of English. Occasionally the
writer would add "(sic)" in parentheses, as if he were not sure of a
certain spelling. Each page was carefully numbered: "#1 of 4," "#2
of 4," and so on.

This note proved to be one of the most vexing and ambiguous
elements of the whole case. Here is what it said:

January 18 1985.
Friday 12:45
Hilton Inn Gainesville

*We have made all our arrangements and now are ready to do
what Page thinks, and I, is the only way we can be together for all
time. The constant interfering with our lives by outsiders is over.
We know that to go on like we have in the past would only eventually turn our love into hate for each other and cause us to eventually seperate. That thought alone is what neither of us can bear to
think about. The love we have had and always had since our eyes
first met in Alaska has been so strong that in just 19 months we
both have proven it more than most people show in a lifetime.
Problems we have had surely but very few of our own—instead
caused by meddling others. The pain Page has gone through because of her family is what makes all we have done in the past
week bearable to me. She was rejected by her family when she
came back from Alaska because she loved someone her family*

didn't approve of. Instead of suporting her and saying we don't understand but are with you—they told her to get rid of me or get out. We went to Texas. Still the interferring (sic) from them and on her father's birthday she was sent money to go home but not to bring me. They were under the impression that we had broken up and were not together, so when she got off the plane her mother took her shopping in Portland, Me. On the way back to Jackson, N.H., she told her mother we were together still. Her mother turned the car around and took all the presents back to the stores. When she finally got to Jackson her father told her to get out and never come back. Her brother told her to get "fucked in the ass" and never wanted to see or hear from her again. She called me in Texas and told me what happened and was getting back to Portland and told me to pick her up in Houston. When she got back home I spent almost four hours with her in my lap talking her through what she was put through. Then we went to Alaska again and worked in the worst possible place for a lonely girl with all these thoughts she never really told me about until last week. The letters from her brother helps to explain what I am writing about. Pressure, rejection, pressure, castigation, pressure and then what took place several weeks ago and more pressure.

Her brother who was "helping" her got to pressuring her thoughts into telling me to leave forever. She couldn't tell him to hurt him or me to hurt me. She kept it all inside and it became too much for her. The final straw for Page came when her brother said we had to get out "by 5:00 P.M. tomorrow" or he would "pull the plug." He left a note telling her to take "the milk, half an onion, cheese, Beck's beer, soup, etc." Which said to Page get everything that will remind me of you and get out of my life. AGAIN.

All our letters to one another have been burned so no one can touch them. All our pictures likewise. She made me promise to burn the home in N.H. to make sure there were no mementos left for anyone to have. It seems that she wants to just disappear so as if never to have been on earth.

In the past week we have talked over plans that were brought up many times when ever she was depressed. At first we would go together and "make them pay." Then it finally came to me going while she waited for me to get back and we'd die together by cremation. Why—because I love her so very much—is the only reason I can think of. More than my own life itself. Sometimes, as I drove up and back, I think she thought I would get up there, do what we wanted and get caught coming back all that time and distance. Only one road out and a fire would attract immediate attention so would be reported quickly. Just a feeling I guess from our meeting on Thursday at noon at her brothers house. She hasn't said much to me since, only that she is ready and was "meditating" the days I was gone. Spiritually she is ready.

You are thinking—this guy is crazy—No I am not. I have functioned like a rational person in every way since we made our plans such as getting motels, eating, driving, selling things in Hartford, buying the shot gun in the event I got stopped on the way back I would use it on myself and not hurt any other innocent person. Page would jump from the bridge in Jacksonville with a car battery tied to her if we couldn't go on together as we had planned. But yes—crazy from love and caring for this lady to want to forever be with her at least mind spirit, and ashes. We are to go together so our ashes cannot be seperated only our bones can be put in two different places as her brother will do. Page says if we died whole he would seperate us by two graves and this way it is impossible.

As I sit here contemplating what is ahead for me is apauling [appalling] (sic) but I have given my word and that is and always has been my bond. Nobody can say about me that once I say I will do something that I've ever not done it. Page knows this and maybe used it. I am not regretting what's been done because if we ever would have called it quits permanently I would have taken all their lives anyway. But now I have to take Page's life with my hands and kill the only love I have left. Page says she needs it that way—her meditation time—directed her. She knows that I will do it and isn't worried that I'll "wimp out" on myself. By not joining her. My word, and she believes in me that much.

Her brother won't be harmed so that he can live with everything for the rest of his life. A pay back for rejecting her and writing that she was "insane" in his journal. Personally I would

*like to wait around and do him but she has made me promise not
to give him the easy way out but to think about it every day. I have
promised to go with her and so we shall.*

*The place we picked out was found by driving around many
miles and it was history, on top of a hill and seemed to be just right
to her. We had two "picnics" there and that is where we made our
plans and promises to one another. She is waiting now and I must
do what I can't believe I'm going to do but I must do for me and
her.*

Here a line is skipped in the note. The last two lines above,
beginning with *"She is waiting now . . ."* are written in a more
hurried and slantwise script, as if dashed off in haste. Several blank
lines follow. The note then resumes:

*Maybe I am crazy at least now for I have taken the life of
the only lady I feel I've ever really been in love with. And I
don't want to die but will just to see if we can be together
again as Page seems to think. It was the most terrible thing,
but feel her love more than ever now it seems.*

The next five words are crossed out, but plainly legible:

I took her in my

The note then continues:

*First I should tell that as we built our cremation it was the
happiest I've seen her in many weeks. She kept talking and had
such an air about her afterwards we talked for about two hours
and just enjoyed each other and hugged and repeated our wedding
vows to one another and hope we are doing what's right for us.*

*When we were ready I took her in my arms and said "Page I
love you." The answer was, "Mike it has always been only you and
I want it to always be that I'm you're very last love."*

*She sat in front of me with me sitting behind and put a choke
hold on and held it for at least two minutes. She never once seemed*

to struggle and when I thought she had expired I released and lowered my arms to hug her. Damn, she started to move and I couldn't do anything else but start rubbing her shoulders and talking to her and in about twenty minutes she was crying in my arms and hoarsely started talking to me and crying too. She said "Mike you promised, you promised"—But I just felt I couldn't anymore. We talked for a little while and then the very last words she said were "Mike I love only you forever" and this time I kept the hold on her until my arms, fingers and body cramped. Lay her down on the blanket and she was still and turning blue. I readied the wood under the platform and she started to jerk a little. I looked at her with the flashlight and this time she wouldn't be coming back but I couldn't stand to see her twitch so hit her with a large stone. That's why her head may be crushed on the right side.

I have decided to rope myself down before I use the shotgun in case I might do the same and fall from our platform. That's the only reason why there may be rope marks on me if they don't burn off or something. The little brown bag are the ashes from her puppy that died in Texas last year. We had it cremated in San Antone and she wanted the ashes sprinkled with us and the present puppy, Chelshea, are the bones with us. I brought her back with me from New Hampshire.

It's time for me to go back up there and finish and be with my love for all times. Page was the most beautiful lady in the world but at times a devil. I feel just because she had so many things working against her—pressure—that finally made us do this last step. If I can spend the rest of my time with her somewhere is all that I can hope for. I loved her

Good bye
D. Mike Daniels
for Page Jennings Daniels

I'm going to start the fire with 21 $100.00 bills for she is just 21 + 16 days.

This extraordinary note, with its proxy signature of Page Jennings Daniels and its dark references to other murders in New

Hampshire *("she made me promise to burn the home in N.H. . . ."* *"We would go together and make them pay . . ."* *"if we ever would have called it quits permanently I would have taken all their lives anyway . . ."),* instantly focused police scrutiny on a ghastly double murder that had occurred twelve days earlier in Pinkham Notch, New Hampshire. Here, summoned to a fire at an old ski lodge called the Dana Inn in the early morning hours of January 16, authorities had found the bodies of Page Jennings's parents, Malcolm Jennings, fifty-four, and his wife, Elizabeth B. Jennings, forty-nine. The couple were discovered dead of multiple stab wounds, tied up with nylon cord in separate bedrooms, gagged before they died. Whoever murdered them had set fire to the inn afterward, hoping to destroy the bodies. As things turned out, however, the corpses suffered only minor smoke damage and were easily identifiable.

As a forensic anthropologist, my work is necessarily focused on the dead more than on the living. I seldom occupy myself professionally with the quirks and foibles of human beings as long as they are alive. When life is extinguished, and the flesh falls away, and the hard frame of the skeleton lies exposed on the laboratory table—that is my hour. But in this case, more than in most others, I was forced to take account of the personalities of the deceased to a far greater degree than is usual for me. Because of the glare of publicity that accompanied this case, the individuals involved stood forth in stark relief, in scores of newspaper articles and television news reports. One man in particular haunted the case. Almost against my will I became acquainted with the life and times of Glyde Earl Meek.

Police had little trouble establishing the true identity of "D. Mike Daniels," the man who signed the suicide note found in the Fiat near the burned cabin. His real name was Glyde Earl Meek, a powerfully built, red-haired Washington State man with a string of arrests for burglary and a prison record. He was an exceptionally athletic specimen, who had captained his college wrestling team at Washington State University. He weighed only 185 pounds in later life, just five pounds more than he had weighed in high school. He was known as a "second-story man" for his burgling feats: he would climb walls and slip into a building through the roof or an upper-story window. His upper arms were exceptionally powerful and his agility was remarkable. Meek "had a crazy body, like a gorilla," a classmate would later recall.

Meek was born in Pasco, Washington, on July 22, 1935, the second of three boys, to Pearl and Joe Meek. Joe Meek, a lineman who worked for several power companies near Seattle, was an abusive husband and beat his wife frequently, according to relatives interviewed by the *Boston Herald* after the murders. "He was a good-for-nothing brute," said Thelma Cole, then seventy-two, Pearl's sister-in-law.

Meek's parents finally divorced. While their mother worked, Glyde Earl and his older brother Alfred and his younger brother Michael were raised by their aunt, Thelma Cole. Cousin Roger Cole said Meek was a scoundrel even as a child. "He was a thief from four, five, six," Cole told reporters from Boston after the murders in New Hampshire. "He had a million-dollar personality and a real gift with folks. It's just that there was a missing link somewhere." Another high school classmate, Ron Jackson, told the *New Hampshire Sunday News* that Meek was "a guy that couldn't live by society's rules. He had a lot of talent but he just couldn't keep it within the system."

Meek entered Pasco High School in the early 1950s, studied there two years and then transferred to Walla Walla High. He was described as "an honor student without effort," who excelled in sports, especially football and wrestling. Once, while skylarking in front of his classmates, he climbed to the top of the Bonneville Power Administration transmission tower in Sacajawea Park, jumped off, grabbed the insulators and swung on them "like a monkey," as one astonished eyewitness put it. Then he swung back to safety as easily as he had swung out. "I thought sure he was grabbing hot wires," said a classmate, Scotty Getchell. "But he did things like that. He was always out for thrills."

Another classmate, Tony Hapler, said Meek "could scale the side of a building, and I saw him do it." It was Hapler who likened Meek to a gorilla. Hapler told the *Manchester Union Leader* that Meek never graduated from college because he was caught stealing a car.

Meek's days at Walla Walla High School were the high-water mark of his success. He rose to become vice-president of the student body. Upon graduation he entered Washington State University on an athletic scholarship but never finished college. He married in 1959, divorced in 1964, leaving his wife with two sons. Meek made no attempt to contact his sons and to this day they do not know they are descended from him.

Meek turned to burglary in the early 1960s, using his strength and agility to break into buildings through the roof. He was caught in 1962 by Art Eggers, Walla Walla's newly appointed chief prosecutor. "Five or six establishments had been burglarized in Walla Walla and also a J. C. Penney Store in Seattle. He used to go in through the tops of stores. He was a hell of a roof burglar," Eggers told reporters.

"When we caught him he had a U-Haul full of about $10,000 in stolen goods—clothing, liquor—from Salt Lake City stores. If you met him in a pub instead of on the battlefield, you'd say he's one of the nicest guys around. I've been at this job a long time and he's about my favorite crook."

Convicted, Meek was sent to Walla Walla State Penitentiary, where he became inmate No. 212104. At first he seemed a model prisoner, starring on the prison football team, but after an unsuccessful escape attempt his prison term was lengthened; he was finally paroled in 1970. The golden middle of his life was nearly over and he had spent eight of his best years in jail. He was now thirty-five.

Meek remarried and started a successful sign business, the Alpine Sign Co. In 1972 Meek's mother, Pearl, committed suicide. She had become an alcoholic and was depressed, relatives said. She drove her Mustang to a ballpark, parked, and left the engine running. Carbon monoxide fumes killed her. At her funeral Meek "wept and wept," friends remembered.

Fred Mielke met Meek, nicknamed "Shorty," as part of a prison volunteer group that helped parolees adjust to life outside. "Shorty was a likable, hard-working guy. If your car had trouble and was on the side of the road, he would be the first person to pull over to help," Mielke said.

When Meek's second marriage fell apart "everything went to hell," Mielke said. A second arrest for burglary followed and Meek was given a one-year sentence. He was paroled in the late 1970s. He then met a woman named Debby Alderfer, from Pennsylvania. Shortly afterward he was arrested while attempting to shoplift a seven-dollar pair of pants. Fearful of being sent back to jail, he fled Spokane, taking Alderfer with him, and went to Tucson, Arizona, where he founded another sign business.

At about this time Meek began using the alias that would appear on the High Springs suicide note: Daniel Mikel Daniels. It was one of about ten false names he used at various times. Meek was a possessive husband who forbade Alderfer to call her parents, ever. For eight years she obeyed him. "I loved him," Alderfer told the *Boston Herald* later. "I felt my life with him was worth it. He had me convinced that if I called [my parents] the line would be traced and he would be sent back to jail."

Many doctors and pathologists tend to look askance at chiropractors, as practicing a profession on the fringes of serious medicine. My own opinion—has no place in this narrative. But I have often-times blessed the impulse that drove Glyde Earl Meek to visit a chiropractor in Arizona in the early 1980s.

This small, chance event would have a crucial bearing on the case, for the chiropractor who treated Meek at the Waldschmitt Clinic in Tucson took six x-rays of Meek's back. These x-rays became the only antemortem pictures of Glyde Earl Meek's living skeleton in existence. As such they were of inestimable value to me. One of the x-ray films showed Meek's upper rib cage. Another, shot rather high, revealed a gold tooth filling. This filling also showed up on dental x-rays of Meek. This small nugget of gold would later prove a crucial piece of evidence.

In 1983 the couple moved to Alaska with the vain hope of panning for gold there. Meek became the caretaker of a vacation lodge at Seal Bay. It was here he met young Page Jennings. It was an encounter that would have the most dreadful consequences for the entire Jennings family.

Page Jennings was a beautiful girl with pale skin and elfin features. She had a quick mind, liked reading and was an expressive writer with a keen sense of humor. Her parents were wealthy and she enjoyed all the advantages of an excellent education and a comfortable upbringing. She seemed destined for a life of happiness and ease.

At the 1,100-student Kennett High School in Conway, New Hampshire, Page Jennings made the National Honor Society and served on the student council, was a homeroom representative, a delegate to the New Hampshire Youth and Government Council. She overcame two knee injuries to throw the javelin for the girls' track team her senior year. These injuries were severe enough to require surgery, and this would later have a crucial bearing on the case. The precise details of the surgical procedure would send me on a wild goose chase that lasted for months and nearly brought me to my wits' end.

Until now life had smiled on Page Jennings. But in her first year at Simmons College in Boston she became acquainted with bitter failure. She studied physical therapy there but did poorly. She failed a difficult but required course in organic chemistry and this failure seems to have shaken her resolve. Page decided to take a year off from school, strike out on her own. She landed a job as a cook at the Seal Bay resort in Alaska where, in June 1983, she met Glyde Earl Meek.

Meek, who was working as a caretaker at the lodge, was instantly smitten with Page Jennings, at least to judge from the wording of the suicide note found near the cabin: "The love we have had and always had since our eyes first met in Alaska has been so strong that in just

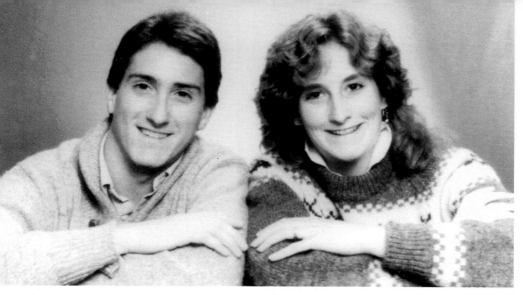

Chris and Page Jennings. Glyde Earl Meek almost certainly intended to murder Chris Jennings, but the young man had flown to New Hampshire for his parents' funeral. (*Courtesy of Chris Jennings.*)

NEW HAMPSHIRE STATE POLICE

WANTED PERSON

Wanted for ___FIRST DEGREE MURDER___   NH RSA ___630:1-a___

NAME   GLYDE EARL MEEK
AGE   49   DOB 07-22-35
RACE   WHITE   SEX MALE
HAIR BROWN - GRAY   EYES BLUE
HEIGHT   5'10"   WEIGHT   185
BUILD   MEDIUM   COMPLEXION   RUDDY/TAN
NATIONALITY   AMERICAN
POB   PASCO, WASHINGTON
FPC   02 OR II 09
      OR OII 10   REFERENCE OTt OR
NCICFPC   PO-02-02-07-09-DO-63-08-10-10
ALIASES   SEE REVERSE SIDE
SCARS AND MARKS

EXTRADITION   NATIONWIDE
NCIC   W 368928092
FBI NUMBER   732 602 B
N. H. BCI NUMBER

GLYDE EARL MEEK IS WANTED FOR THE MURDERS OF MALCOLM AND ELIZABETH JENNINGS OF JACKSON, NEW HAMPSHIRE. THE MURDERS TOOK PLACE IN THE JENNINGS RESIDENCE ON THE EVENING OF JANUARY 15 OR THE EARLY MORNING HOURS OF JANUARY 16, 1985. THE BODIES OF THE VICTIMS WERE LOCATED BY FIREMEN IN THE PROCESS OF EXTINGUISHING A FIRE AT THE JENNINGS RESIDENCE. THE CAUSE OF THE FIRE HAS BEEN DEEMED ARSON. BOTH VICTIMS DIED AS A RESULT OF MULTIPLE STAB WOUNDS.

MEEK HAS USED MULTIPLE ALIASES, DIFFERENT DATES OF BIRTH AND SOCIAL SECURITY NUMBERS. HE SHOULD BE CONSIDERED ARMED AND DANGEROUS.

PLEASE SEE REVERSE SIDE FOR MORE DETAILS.

COLONEL PAUL F. O'LEARY
     DIRECTOR
TEL. #603-271-3636

CASE   I-85-004
DATE   06-21-85
NBR   85-016W

A wanted poster for Glyde Earl Meek, printed five months after his death.

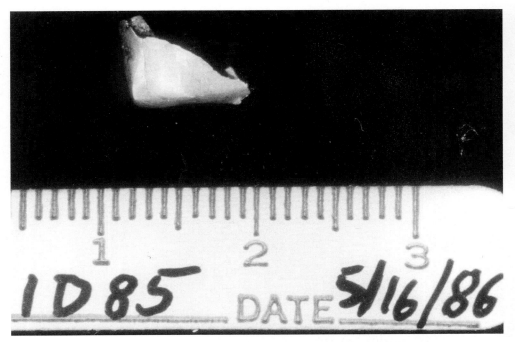

The gold inlay from the tooth of Glyde Earl Meek. Originally missed by investigators, this crucial piece of evidence was later recovered when earth from the scene was resifted through a finer-meshed screen.

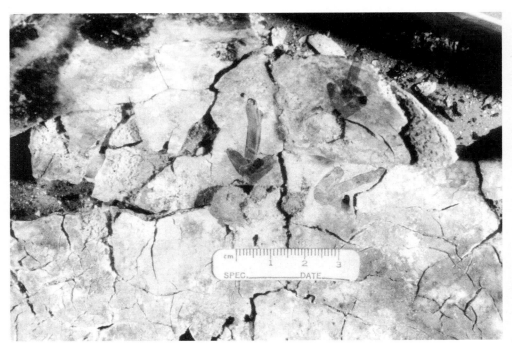

Shotgun pellets (arrows) stuck to the inside of Glyde Earl Meek's braincase.

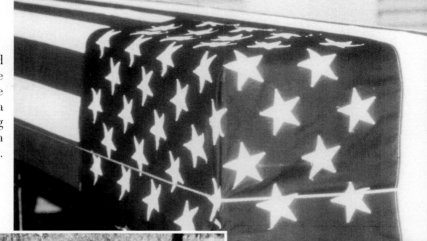

A flag-draped
transfer case
containing the
remains of a
soldier missing
in action in
Vietnam.

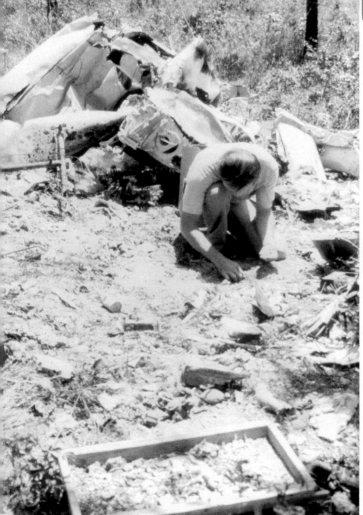

Searching for cremated
dental and skeletal
evidence at the crash
site of a single-engine
aircraft.

Dr. Robert Benfer and I examine the bones of Pizarro at the Cathedral of San Agustín in Lima, Peru. *(Photo courtesy of Margaret Maples.)*

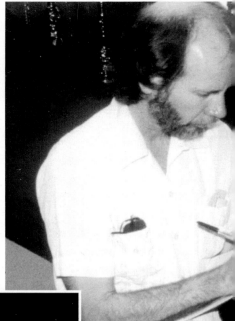

The skull of Don Francisco Pizarro, conqueror of Peru, assassinated Sunday, June 26, 1541.

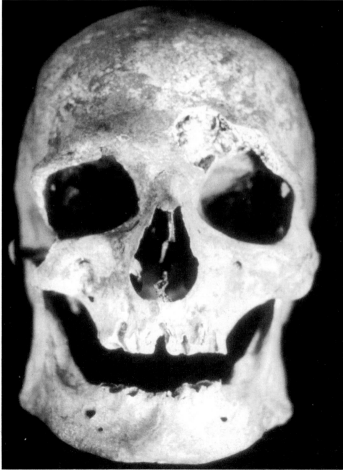

A mock sword shows the path of one of Pizarro's many wounds.

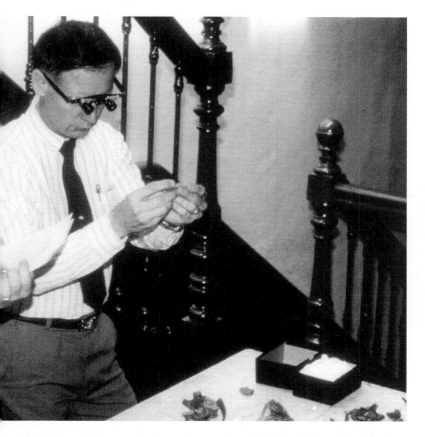

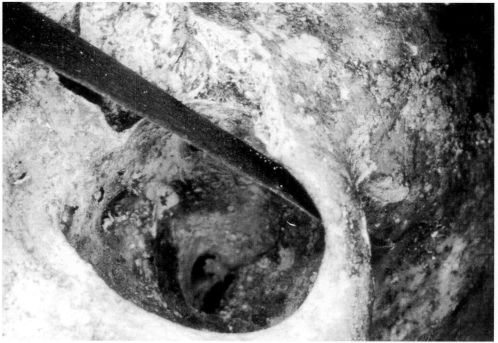

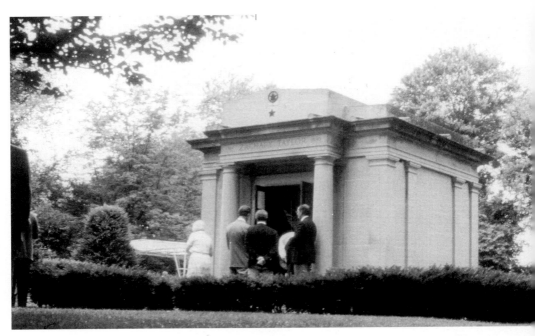

The tomb of Zachary Taylor in Louisville, Kentucky. *(Photo courtesy of Arlene Albert.)*

Perforations in the leaden inner casket of Zachary Taylor were caused by oxidation. *(Photo courtesy of Arlene Albert.)*

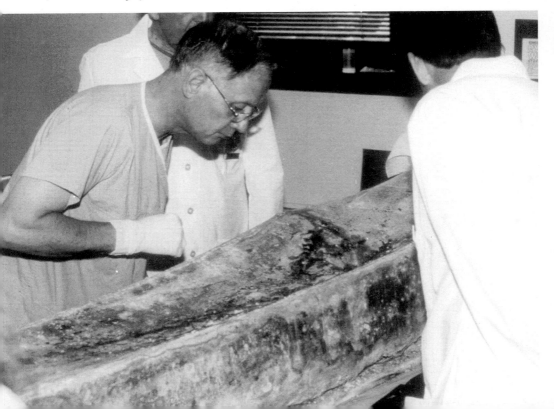

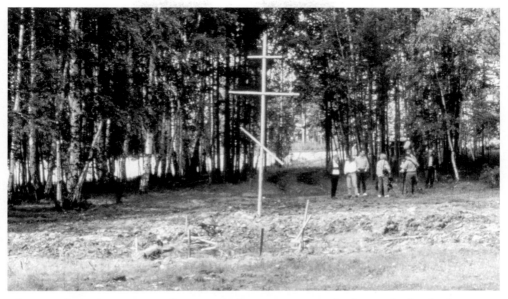

The site where the remains of Tsar Nicholas II were unearthed is marked today by a makeshift Russian Orthodox cross.

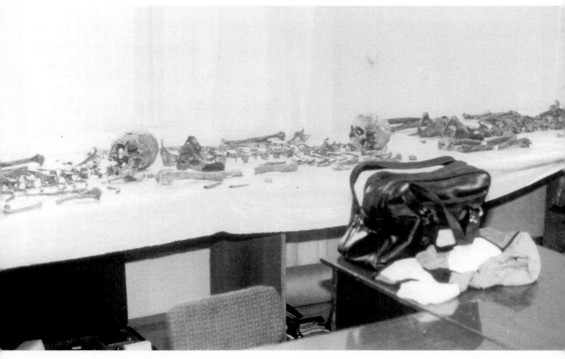

The bones of the Tsar, his family and servants, arranged on tables at the forensic institute of Ekaterinburg. From left to right in this view are the remains of Dr. Eugene Botkin, Grand Duchess Olga and Tsar Nicholas II.

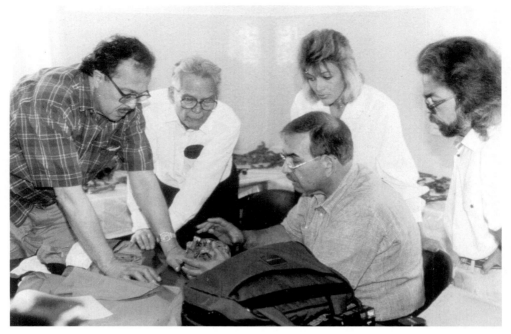

Dr. Lowell Levine explains the dental evidence to (left to right) Dr. Michael Baden, Dr. William Goza, Tatyana Kondrashova and a Russian expert.

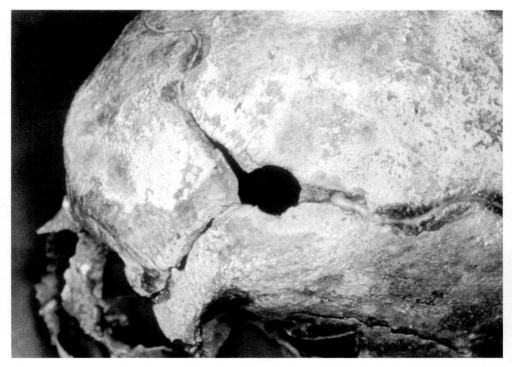

The entrance wound in the top left side of Dr. Botkin's skull. All the bullets recovered and all the bullet wounds observed were consistent with .32-caliber ammunition.

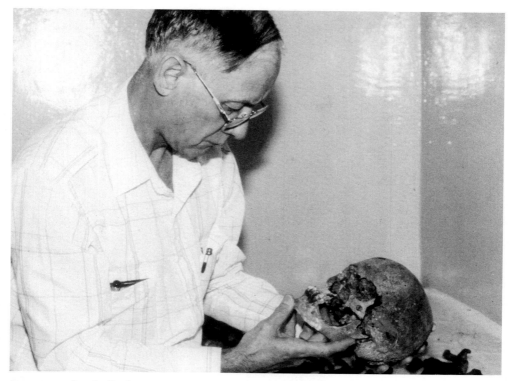

I examine the skull of
Tsar Nicholas II.

The cranium of
Body No. 5, showing
the missing portions
of the face. This was
the youngest skull in
the group, but it is
still too old to be
Anastasia's.

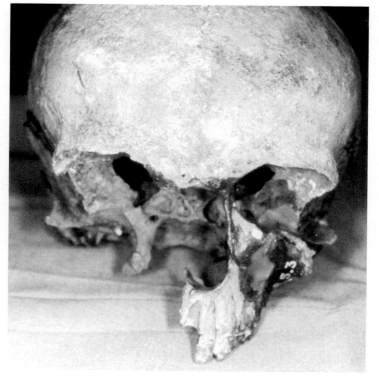

The entrance wound in the top left side of the head of Body No. 6. This skull may have belonged to the Grand Duchess Tatiana.

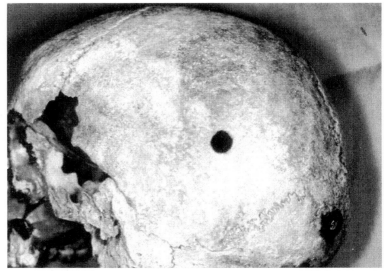

The skull of Grand Duchess Titiana.

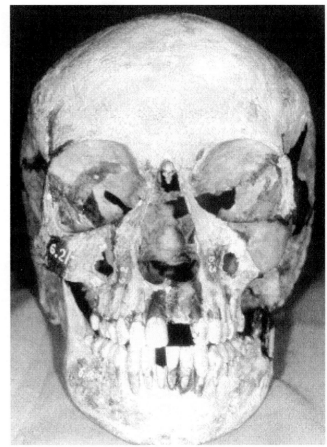

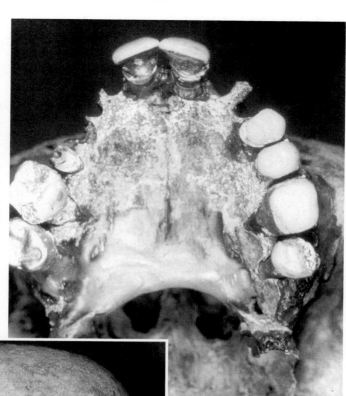

Tsarina Alexandra's upper jaw and numerous gold and porcelain crowns and platinum crowns, and dental restorations. This exquisite dental work was the first sign to the excavators that the occupants of the burial pit were royalty.

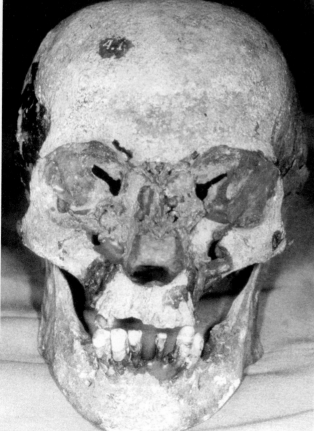

The skull of Tsar Nicholas II.

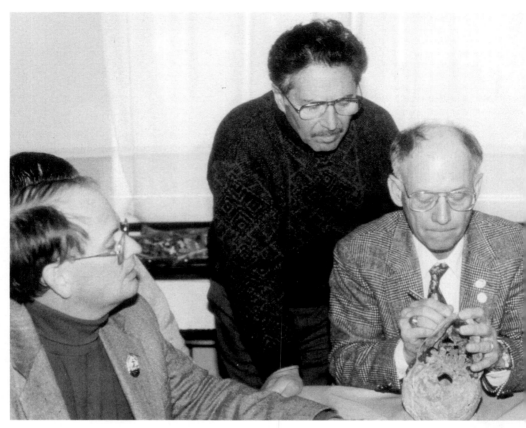

Dr. William Hamilton and Dr. Alexander Melamud look on as I extract a tooth for later DNA analysis. *(Photo courtesy of Margaret Maples.)*

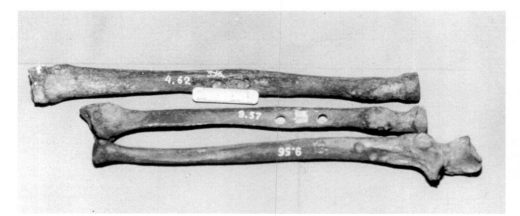

A radius (above in the photograph) from the arm associated with Body No. 4 (Tsar Nicholas) is clearly larger than the radius and ulna now associated with Body No. 9 (the footman, Trupp). It ought to be shorter. I therefore believe that these radii have gotten mixed up, and that the Tsar will be served in death, as he was in life, by the arms of his faithful footman.

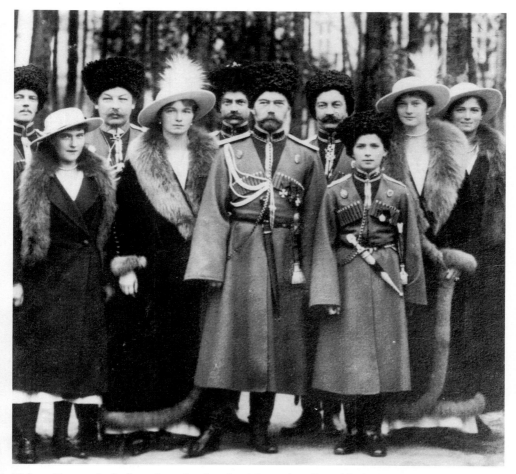

Taken 21 months before their deaths, the relative heights of (left to right) Anastasia, Olga, Tsar Nicholas II, Alexei, Tatiana and Marie can be seen. *(Photo courtesy of Beineke Library, Yale University.)*

The family relationship between Tsarina Alexandra and Prince Phillip, the Duke of Edinburgh. Mitochondrial DNA is passed on through the female line and remains the same, generation after generation.

Albert of Saxe-Coburg = Queen Victoria

Louis IV of Hesse = Alice

Victoria = Louis of Battenberg

Alice = Prince Andrew of Greece

Philip Mountbatten (Duke of Edinburgh)

Alexandra = Nicholas II

Olga Tatiana Marie Anastasia Alexei

RELATIONSHIP OF ALEXANDRA AND HER CHILDREN TO PRINCE PHILIP MOUNTBATTEN (DUKE OF EDINBURGH)

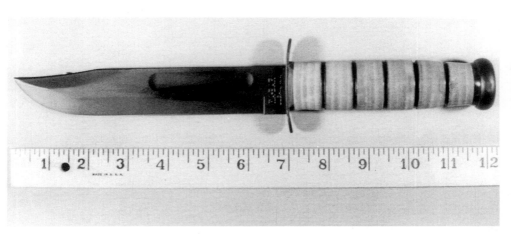

A Ka-Bar knife similar to that used by Danny Rolling in the Gainesville student murders.

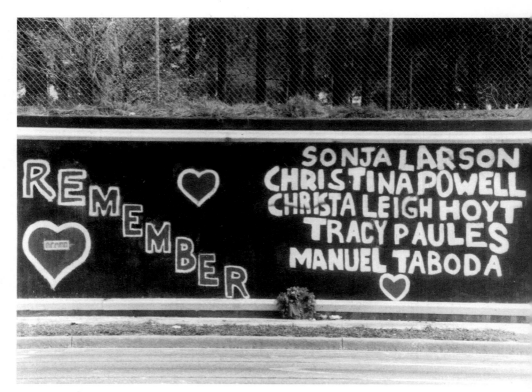

The wall near my office in Gainesville, memorializing the five students murdered in Gainesville in 1990. Rolling pleaded guilty the first day of his trial. A jury recommended the death penalty. *(Photo courtesy of Michael Warren.)*

19 months we both have proven it more than most people show in a lifetime."

Meek's third wife, Debby Alderfer, took a dimmer view of the relationship. She later told the *Boston Herald* that Page "had a lot of problems," and that Meek "seemed to want to help her out, protect her. . . . He became obsessed with her."

Page seemed to enjoy the attentions of the older man. Meek took her on nature trips and, much later, she rapturously described seeing an American bald eagle for the first time in Alaska, on a trip with a friend she called "Mike," who was obviously Meek.

"When one thinks of the American bald eagle, visions of thundering, snowcapped mountains and rushing rivers in Canada, Alaska and the northern states invade the mind," Page wrote. "Keep your eyes skyward and your ears open. Maybe one day you'll see the magnificent bird overhead."

In the fall of 1983 the unlikely trio left Alaska together. Eventually an unhappy Debby Alderfer saw she was no longer wanted and bowed out. "I'm not bitter now," she told reporters later. "I was hoping he would find some kind of happiness, but I guess he didn't."

In October 1983, Page took Meek to visit her parents in Jackson, New Hampshire. The visit was an unmitigated disaster. The whole family was shocked and repelled by the vagabond, middle-aged, uncouth man their daughter had fallen in love with. To the Jenningses, Meek appeared a creature from another world, a man whose past was as murky as his future was dim. Page's older brother, Chris Jennings, was openly disgusted by Meek and did nothing to hide his contempt.

"This guy had no history, no ambition. She could have done a lot better," Christopher Jennings later said to reporters.

Determined to stay together, the couple headed south in the last months of 1983, moving into a modern duplex in Palm Harbor, Texas, near the town of Rockport. Page landed a job as a sportswriter at a local weekly paper, the *Rockport Pilot*, where she worked from December 1983 to April 1984. A coworker, Bobbie Drennon, recalled that at least once Page Jennings came to work with bruises on her face. Page admitted she had had a fight with Meek. *"Page was the most beautiful lady in the world but at times a devil,"* Meek later wrote in the suicide note.

She stayed in touch with her parents, who made it clear they still loved her but despised Meek. In the spring of 1984 she and Meek decided to return to Alaska. Page left a good-bye note for her co-workers, using a quote from D. H. Lawrence.

> *Dear Pilot friends:*
>
> *I leave you with these words of wisdom. There is no point in work unless it absorbs you like an absorbing game. If it doesn't absorb you, it isn't fun, don't do it. "All that we have while we live is life. If you don't live during your life, all you are is a piece of dung." Fare ye well, Page.*

But the relationship was beginning to erode and crumble. Fewer than six months after returning to Alaska, Meek and Jennings headed south again. They broke up in Seattle and Page returned to Rockport, Texas, in September 1984, then went back to New England. She visited a psychiatrist, then decided to accompany her brother Christopher to Gainesville, Florida, where he had landed a job with the *Gainesville Sun.*

Page Jennings got a job as a waitress at the Stacks restaurant in the Gainesville downtown Holiday Inn. Soon afterward, around December 4, 1984, Glyde Earl Meek appeared and persuaded Page to let him move in with her, sharing her bedroom in the apartment where she was living with her brother Chris.

Chris Jennings was disgusted and infuriated. Not only was the loathsome Meek back in his sister's life again, he was squatting under the selfsame roof now. Chris was on the threshold of a new career and was trying to help his sister get her life straightened out. But Meek wouldn't let go, and Page seemed unable to find the backbone to break up with him. Life in the little apartment became unendurable for all three. Page found herself vacillating hopelessly between two men who detested each other.

"It always seemed like, when there was a conflict, Page ended up getting hurt. I was trying to find a way to make him feel hurt. I didn't like him because he was pulling Page one way and my parents were pulling her another," Chris Jennings said later.

"Her brother who was 'helping' her got to pressuring her thoughts into telling me to leave forever. She couldn't tell him to hurt him or me to hurt me. She kept it all inside and it became too much for her," Meek had written in the longer suicide note.

"She was a real nice girl but she had a lot of problems," a waiter named John Hughes told reporters after the deaths. "I think she wanted to get away from the guy, but she didn't know how and was scared to."

Another worker at the Stacks restaurant, Kenneth Denman, recounted afterward how he saw Meek several times when he came to pick up Page after her shift at the Holiday Inn. He described Meek as "rough-looking." He remembered how Meek would sit in a booth and drink coffee, wearing a red and white baseball hat with the word "Page" stenciled across the bill.

Throughout late December and early January, Meek came and went on mysterious business trips. Police have traced his movements to Louisiana, Texas and Jacksonville, Florida, where he bought the blue Fiat later found in the field beside the burned cabin. He seems to have stolen another Fiat, this one painted silver, in Corpus Christi, Texas, on January 5.

Page decided not to go home for Christmas 1984. Her parents were bitterly disappointed. This decision may have played a part in the tragic denouement, now only days away.

On January 5, 1985, after an ugly three-way quarrel, Page Jennings and Glyde Earl Meek moved out of the apartment she shared with her brother Chris. Chris told her she would have to leave unless she renounced Meek, in which case she would be welcome to stay.

Page chose Meek. The couple took a room at the Gator Court Motel in Gainesville. Meek rented a storage space in a mini-warehouse named Atkins Storage. On January 11, Page went back to collect her half of the apartment deposit. It was the last time her brother saw her alive.

Now Meek headed north alone, on an errand of murder. On January 12 he booked a room at a motel in Brattleboro, North Carolina. The next night he checked into the Bridgeport Motor Inn in Connecticut.

On January 14, Meek was seen in Hartford, Connecticut, attempting to pawn some jewelry. The pawnbroker recalled that Meek had said the jewelry belonged to his daughter, who had died in a skiing accident. Later in the same conversation he switched stories, saying his daughter had died in a car accident.

Matters now moved to mortal conclusions. On January 16, in New Hampshire, Malcolm and Betty Jennings were found murdered in their blazing hotel. They had been tied up with nylon rope in separate bedrooms before being stabbed to death. Their son Chris was notified by police and left for New Hampshire immediately. This act of filial piety probably saved his life, because police later found a second suicide note, also dated January 18 and signed by Meek, in Chris Jennings's apartment.

In his first suicide note, found near the scene, Meek seemed to describe the anxieties of traveling up to New Hampshire to murder Page's parents and setting fire to their inn.

> In the past week we have talked over plans that were brought up many times when ever she was depressed. At first we would go together and "make them pay." It finally came to me going while she waited for me to get back and we'd die together by cremation. . . . Sometimes, as I drove up and back, I think she thought I would get up there, do what we wanted and get caught coming back all that time and distance. Only one road out and a fire would attract immediate attention so would be reported quickly. . . .

Later, after the burned cabin and the skeletons were discovered near High Springs, police visited Chris Jennings's apartment seeking evidence. They found a desperate message from Chris to Page taped to the door of the apartment. Written moments after Chris had been notified of the murders of his parents and was en route to New Hampshire, the note gave Page three emergency telephone numbers to call. The rest of the message read:

PAGE!
I *REALLY* NEED YOU!
LOVE,
CHRIS

But there was a heavy scrawl in another hand defacing this note. The "you!" at the end of the first line had been crossed out and a huge **NO!** had been scrawled over it and underlined many times.

Inside the apartment, on two sheets of *Gainesville Sun* stationery in the same handwriting as that used in the long suicide note found in the Fiat, Meek had written his last, angry message to Chris Jennings. This note spoke clearly of the New Hampshire murders, referring to the older Jenningses as "Mal" and "Betty":

Friday 18 Jan 1985

This and the note telling Page to take the "eggs, milk, flour, onions, cheese—etc did it Bucko. We are together now always and forever. Mike.

"Right will prevail" as you wrote in your scheeming letter to Page in Alaska about taking the bus, or flying, or riding down to Seattle or riding down to Texas and then pretending to go home for a couple weeks. You bastard—!

"Daniels is a dead man" if he comes here, you wrote.

You live with it all now, Bucko—Mal, Betty and us. Meddling fools.

Page is so bitter that this is the only way she can see how we can be together forever. Cremation.

Death in 10,000 Fragments

Call the police—they have some letters and information for you or what-ever.

This second note is unsigned, save for the name "Mike," after the first paragraph, presumably derived from Meek's alias, Daniel Mikel Daniels, the same name he used in the second, longer suicide note.

Both suicide notes are dated January 18 and it appears the old abandoned cabin was set on fire that day. The Jenningses were buried in New Hampshire on January 19, and Chris Jennings spoke the eulogy. He still believed his sister was alive. "I'm sure she's just off playing and will be devastated when she hears the news," he said to reporters.

On January 28 the fire-wasted cabin and the calcined skeletons were discovered near High Springs. Two days later the remains were delivered over to me for examination.

My feelings upon seeing the thousands of commingled bone fragments pour out of the vinyl body bag in a chalky cascade are impossible to convey. Nothing in the entire range of my professional experience approached the daunting complexities of this problem. These bones had not merely been broken; they had been ground up as if by some grim apothecary's pestle. How could I hope to make sense of them?

Although the powdery and jumbled condition of the remains before me looked hopeless, there were some encouraging aspects of the case. True, the medical examiner's investigator had collected all the bones in a single bag, but before this happened Alachua County Sheriff's Department investigators had taken good, clear photographs of the crime scene. The department provided me with large, clear blowups of these photographs, nearly three feet high and very detailed. In them the disposition of the remains, precisely as they were found, could be seen with considerable clarity.

There was the wire mesh, there was the shotgun barrel, there were the bone fragments, lying in distinct little heaps, just as they had been found, untouched. Some of the larger pieces before me could be assigned to one or the other of the two piles. It soon became clear that we were dealing with a pair of adult human remains, one male, one female, both Caucasoid. The female was very likely between the ages of twenty and twenty-five years. The male was probably between forty-five and sixty years of age.

The brainpan of the male skeleton had several lumps of heavy buckshot, molten and fused to the inner lining of the skull. There were minute traces of lead on the male lower jaw. Clearly a shotgun barrel had been inserted into the mouth of the male and the weapon had been fired before the fire consumed both his body and the wooden parts of the gun that killed him. I have already mentioned how the Ithaca shotgun barrel, with its breech welded shut by the fire, was found near the feet of the male remains.

In the days before x-rays, the means of identifying unknown dead bodies were few and fallible. Confronted with a badly decomposed body or some skeletal remains, you could only identify the deceased by his or her possessions: clothes, jewelry, personal effects. The clothing of Glyde Earl Meek and Page Jennings had been found in the trunk of the Fiat parked nearby. Not a shred of fabric, apart from a small swatch of old, charred burlap unrelated to the skeletons, was found in the ruins of the cabin. Nor were any personal effects found amid the skeletal remains.

The long, rambling suicide notes found in the Fiat and in Chris Jennings's apartment in Gainesville had an air of the theatrical about them. Their extraordinary length was unusual. The fact that they were signed only by Meek/Daniels was odd—why hadn't Page Jennings contributed to the notes, or at least signed them? The fervent protestations of undying love that she supposedly made to Meek just before he choked her sounded false, coming from a girl who was deeply soul-divided between her lover and her family. Her supposed joy at beholding her funeral pyre seemed too ridiculous for words. There was no record of Meek's ever having checked into the Gainesville Hilton Hotel, where he allegedly wrote one note. The bungled strangling, followed by the brutal braining with a rock, jarred sharply with the tender sentiments of romance Meek insists he shared with Page.

My study is of bones, not souls. Suicide notes lie outside my purview. Even today I am bound to say that I do not attach the psychological importance to this note that others have. But I freely confess it is a very strange thing.

Others were piqued more strongly by the note. Dr. Curtis Mertz, a well-known forensic dentist working on the case, went so far as to ask several experts to study it: a forensic psychiatrist, an experienced psychologist and a graphologist, or handwriting expert, with a psychological background. All three believed the note was false. "Artificial," "not believable," "fishy," "too theatrical," were some of their comments. One asked openly the question that bothered us all: *"Why didn't Page Jennings write the note?"*

Here are some of the psychological conclusions that emerged from the note:

> The male has a narcissistic histrionic personality, illusions of grandeur and great self-importance, very self-centered with unrealistic goals, is in love with himself, has a fantasy of IDEAL LOVE, shows increased confusion as the letter progresses and may have had a major depression in the past.

> The female: has a passive aggressive personality, lacks self-confidence and is dependent on others, has a separation anxiety. She wants to get back with her family. I THINK THIS IS A FAKE SUICIDE NOTE.

The graphologist agreed, with some reservations:

> The male is a person able to lie and deceive, is threatened by his insecurities, tends to put off things. His ego comes through like a club. Has a clever demeanor. He is bluffing in the last page about the fire. It is possible, but not likely, that this is a real suicide note.

Thus were planted the seeds of doubt. What if the skeletons in the cabin were not those of Glyde Earl Meek and Page Jennings?

What if the pair were alive and the murder-suicide pact were staged, with two substitute bodies? More sinister still, what if Page Jennings had indeed been murdered by a jealous lover fearful of losing her? What if Meek had covered his tracks by substituting another male corpse to lie beside her body in the burning shack? Was all the purple passion about wanting to be with her forever, mingling his ashes with hers for all eternity—were all those sighs the clever counterfeitings of a cunning murderer? Whose bones were these that lay upon my table?

More mischief was to come. A forensic anthropologist can usually find a firm footing in the study of the remains themselves, their careful analysis and comparison. Bones may riddle us, but they never lie. Yet in the Meek-Jennings case even this calm, clear haven of physical evidence became treacherous ground, swept by ambushes and betrayals.

The first of these I call "Meek's Last Joke." This accident, more than anything else, turned what should have been a straightforward case of identification into a Machiavellian hall of mirrors, an ingenious plot to mislead the investigators. It revolved around a single tooth. Meek would have laughed, to know what misery it caused Dr. Mertz and me.

When the police were searching for medical records and tracing the movements, not only of Page Jennings but especially of Glyde Earl Meek, they found a car that had belonged to him in the care of one of his former girlfriends. She allowed investigators to search the car and in the car they found a matchbox. In the matchbox was a healthy normal tooth belonging to Glyde Earl Meek. In the tooth was a filling that clearly identified the tooth as Meek's, when compared with his dental x-rays.

Another loose tooth had been found among the ashes of the cabin and clearly identified as Meek's. So the fear took shape that Meek had pulled his own teeth to salt a death scene with identifiable evidence from his own mouth. This second tooth, found in a matchbox hundreds of miles away, was the germ from which a plague of doubt would spread. From this point onward there gradually took shape a blind, irrational mistrust of anything found among the ashes that could be identified as Meek's. Such objects, it was reasoned, proved nothing. Meek could have put them there to deceive us. Meek would do anything to throw us off the scent. He would yank out his own teeth and cast them into the flames.

What wasn't found was almost as important as what was. Meek's dental x-rays showed a prominent gold filling in his lower jaw. Dental gold has a high melting point. Even though the cabin had burned like a torch, the heat would have been insufficient to melt this gold filling. Yet the gold filling was nowhere to be found. The earth had been sifted through ⅛-inch mesh screens and it had not turned up. Thus we were being whipsawed from two directions: the tooth that was found after the fire proved nothing; the filling that was lost proved everything.

But these difficulties paled by comparison with the examination of the female's upper jaw. Here we had a very badly burned, calcined, chalk-white palate with many of the teeth still attached. Unfortunately it was so small that it seemed to belong to a midget. If you measure a normal palate in a small, unburned female skull, you will find it is about 49–50 millimeters across, something in that neighborhood. This tiny, burned palate was only 43 millimeters wide —fifteen percent smaller than normal. How could we reconcile this miniature palate with Page Jennings, a fully grown twenty-one-year-old woman? Dr. Mertz told me what I already knew: we had a problem.

The third doubt that bedeviled us was the female tibia. Page Jennings, you may recall, had injured a knee at age seventeen, throwing the javelin in high school. She underwent surgery to repair this injury. The surgeon no longer had the relevant x-rays, but she assured me that she had made two incisions in the surface of the tibia and attached the tendon through them. This is called a Hauser procedure, and it leaves definite and characteristic marks: the bone is cut through in two small parallel rectangles and these rectangles remain visible, even after they have healed over, for the rest of the patient's life.

I had the New Hampshire surgeon sketch the rectangles in pencil on a sample tibia I took up to her. I still have it today. She drew two rectangles on it in pencil at the precise spots where, she insisted, she had cut into Page Jennings's kneebone. Seeing them, I was deeply perplexed. I knew very well that, on the burned and painstakingly reconstructed portion of female tibia that was lying on a table at the C. A. Pound Human Identification Laboratory in Gainesville, there was absolutely no trace of these surgical scars. I had carefully reassembled this five-inch portion of tibia from thirty-six separate fragments of bone, x-rayed it and pored over it for days. And the scars *should have been there,* if indeed the burned bone belonged to Page Jennings.

These doubts were incorporated in our report to the New Hampshire state attorney general's office in 1985. To my vast annoyance, Attorney General Stephen Merrill released all the doubtful points to the press immediately, and the media had a field day. The skeletons in the shack were bogus! Glyde Earl Meek was still alive! Page Jennings couldn't be identified with the female remains in the shack! A murderer and his love-struck girlfriend were still on the loose! Meek was placed on the FBI's "10 Most Wanted" list and his photograph was circulated to law enforcement agencies all over America.

These suspicions grew like weeds. The whole case was taking on a perverse life of its own, a life after death in which skeletons rose up and scampered away on miraculously healed legs; adult jaws shrank to the size of children's; teeth flew out of mouths, and a prominent gold filling somehow evaporated to atoms. To this day, I imagine, there are people in New Hampshire who believe Glyde Earl Meek committed the perfect triple murder and is cavorting around the country as you read these lines, laughing at the law.

These proceedings filled me with chagrin. At the same time I purposed, not without some anger, to get to the bottom of this endlessly mocking case, no matter how long it might take me.

It took me and my students another full year. I doubt if, within the whole history of forensic anthropology, a pair of skeletons has been puzzled over and put back together with such painstaking slowness, such infinite care, as the remains from the burned shack in High Springs. Whenever I had a spare moment in 1985 and 1986, I would return to these two skeletons, cautiously matching up fragments, one by one, bit by bit. Today these remains are kept in two cardboard boxes in the C. A. Pound Human Identification Laboratory, numbered 1C85 and 1D85.

In those days I was still occupying rooms at the Florida Museum of Natural History. At that time in my lab we didn't have huge tables to work on. The expansion of other activities in the museum was cramping me. So I used two counter tops, manufactured at a Florida state prison with convict labor, each one thirty inches deep by eight feet long. One counter top I used for unsorted material. The other I divided into two areas: "His" and "Hers."

Very quickly we could confirm that we had two individuals, no more. Furthermore we could rely on those beautiful, enormous, detailed crime scene photographs taken by the Alachua County sheriff's office, which pretty well indicated that we were dealing with two individuals lying side by side. The dog and squirrel bones presented no great problems. We were able to winnow them out fairly early on. Some types of dog teeth do indeed resemble human "canine" teeth at first glance, but there are distinctive ridges that mark dog teeth clearly and no forensic anthropologist could long be deceived by them.

It was also clear that we were dealing with bones that had burned inside of bodies because of the tremendous twisting and warping and checkering and very characteristic breakage of the bones.

I ask the reader's patience for taking up again a subject I have touched on earlier, that is, the idiosyncrasies of burned bones. But it is essential that you have a clear picture of this process if you are to accompany me in the investigation that follows. Naked bones that are burned in a fire look much different from bones that are enclosed and burned inside a body. Bones burned as bones, and not as part of a body, react differently under fire than do bones encased in tissue with high fat content and other fluids. In some ways it may be considered as the difference between frying a joint of meat in a pan of bacon grease, as opposed to cooking a naked bone in a hot dry oven. Bones burned naked, without the surrounding flesh, go through the same color changes as bones in fresh bodies. They blacken, gray and whiten. They will shrink, but often not as much, and they don't warp and distort themselves as much; nor do the bone surfaces change and degrade in the manner we see in bones burned inside bodies.

When bones inside bodies are burned they change color, as the surrounding flesh sizzles and melts away. These transformations happen quickest around the joints, where the skin, soft tissue and muscles are thinner. Here the transformation begins earliest, but eventually it will overtake the whole skeleton if the fire is allowed to burn.

The bone begins to change from its normal color, a creamy white-yellow, to a darker yellow as fats from the surrounding tissue are baked in. Then, as the fire continues to burn, this dark yellow gradually yields to black. The black represents the organic substances of the bone, which have been carbonized. Finally, if these black, carbonized bones remain amid the flames, even the last organic residues are burned away. In these final stages, the color of the bone gradually fades from black to very dark gray, to gray, to light gray and finally to white. When all of the organic constituents of the bone have been burned away completely, leaving only the inorganic portions—calcium carbonate and other salts of organic material—the bones are pure white. Such are the "calcined bones" you encounter in Gothic novels. My point is, fire and bone interact in very predictable ways, going through a clearly visible series of changes, changes which can be pinpointed by color and texture.

As the fire reaches the bone, definite changes occur. Each bone seems to react differently, according to the thickness of the compact bone composing it. Some surfaces begin to "checker" and break into tiny cubes which may or may not separate from one another.

If it does not pain you too much to imagine your leg on fire, I will tell you that, once your flesh is consumed, the surfaces of your tibia—your shinbone—will begin to split into a crisscross checkerboard pattern. This is because the surface of your tibia is relatively thin.

Now if you don't mind, let the fire move up and consume your thigh. The thighbone is called the femur and here the burn pattern of the surface is completely different, because the outer layer of the femur is thicker. Instead of checkerboards, your thighbone will crackle up into little crescent moons as the fire makes its way through the flesh and begins to gnaw at the bone. Bits may fall off, but they can often be glued back on in the laboratory because of their shape: curved, not right-angled. It's all very distinctive. So the fragments of a burned tibia look very different from the fragments of a burned femur. In my laboratory I was able to divide many small bits of burned bone into checkerboards and crescent moons, and gradually fit these pieces back together into tibias and femurs. In this particular case I was able to reconstruct a large portion of the burned female's tibia out of thirty-six small fragments.

I cannot hope to convey the immense, fatiguing and yet fascinating task of reassembling those fragments. We used Duco cement—model airplane glue—to put the bones back together because it does not expand when subjected to moisture, and because you can always dissolve it with acetone if you make a mistake. I challenged my students to attack these bones and carefully monitored their reconstructions. When I agreed, the reconstruction stood. When I disagreed—out poured the acetone.

Often the fragments were so frail that they had to be splinted after they were glued together. The female's reconstructed tibia is a very twisty thing now: it has a curled flake coming off it like a bean sprout; but when it was part of the living bone, this wild curl lay flat and straight and matched up very nicely with the cavity beneath it. Blame the fire for splitting it and blistering it up. Such are the idiosyncrasies of burned bones.

To sum up a year and a half's work in a single paragraph: We looked for fragments that could be identified as coming from particular bones. We carefully gauged the thickness of the bone walls. We closely measured the curvature of fragments, which indicated the circumference of a certain bone shaft. We looked carefully at the size of the cavity within the shaft as opposed to the thickness of the walls of the shaft. We scrutinized the shapes of joint surfaces and kept an eye out for the special protuberances that indicated muscle attachment. Color was our ally. We always looked at color, the shades of color a bone goes through as it is burning: cream, dark yellow, black, dark gray, gray, light gray, white. Neighboring colors and neighboring textures helped us figure out the coherence of neighboring bones and fragments, what went next to what.

You must not imagine that at the end of our labors we had anything resembling a pair of fully articulated skeletons. Rather, we were trying to reconstruct certain large, significant, verifiable bones that would correspond to x-rays taken of Page Jennings and Glyde Earl Meek before death.

One by one the baffling difficulties and discrepancies yielded to patient endeavor. The first riddle, the tiny female palate, so small it seemed to belong to a midget, was proved to be an adult palate shrunken by fire. I was able to demonstrate that fire shrinks and compresses bones by a factor of twenty to twenty-five percent. The teeth in this palate matched Page Jennings's dental x-rays. It was her palate.

Then came the unscarred tibia. If Page Jennings had undergone radical knee surgery at age seventeen, why didn't the female kneebone show traces of it? When I went back to the New Hampshire surgeon and asked her—very diplomatically of course—to give me copies of her surgical records relating to Page Jennings, I found that she had not used the bone-cutting Hauser procedure, at all, but instead a gentler method known as the Goldthwait procedure, which did not involve cutting into the bone. The surgeon had simply forgotten which type of surgical procedure she had used, but her case records were clear and unequivocal: Goldthwait, not Hauser. This regrettable lapse of memory had cost us months of desperate groping. Now, with the surgical records before me, this riddle was solved.

Page Jennings didn't have surgical scars on her tibia because the surgeon had never cut into the tibia. The surgeon finally agreed with my identification.

With these discrepancies overcome, the rest of the female bones fell into place rather neatly. Her left humerus, or upper-arm bone, closely matched predeath x-rays of Page Jennings's arm, right down to a tiny bone bubble that looked like a capital letter A with two crossbars. There was also a distinctive dome-shaped formation, as well as areas of density, that were recognizable and congruent— almost mathematically so. Page Jennings's deltoid tuberosity—a bump or area of roughened bone where the deltoid muscle attaches to the humerus—was identical in the female humerus found at the burned shack. The maverick fragment of fibula that had somersaulted out of the fire and was only charred at one tip matched up perfectly with x-rays of Page Jennings's left fibula. It became one of our most conclusive pieces of evidence.

To those who, from mischief, fantasy or fond hope, imagine that Page Jennings somehow walked away from that terrible fire, I can only reply: if she did, then she managed to walk away without a major bone in her left leg, her upper left arm, and her palate. That may sound harsh, but in this case the truth had to be used as a blunt instrument. That fibula, that humerus and that palate are today in the C. A. Pound Human Identification Laboratory, and they are all incontestably hers.

Now Meek: from the outset Meek's powerful, stop-at-nothing personality had animated this case diabolically. Page Jennings was merely his plaything and possession. By his own admission in the suicide note, he had murdered her parents in New Hampshire and set the inn on fire. He had then strangled Page, not once but twice, and crushed her skull with a rock. If the evidence in this case were false, it was Meek who had falsified it. If the bones in the shack were not his, he had nevertheless put them there. If this dismal tale were ever to have an ending, it rested with me to determine whether the male skeleton retrieved from the burned cabin belonged to Glyde

Earl Meek or not. Did that buckshot-spattered, fire-cracked brain-pan belong to a self-proclaimed murderer or to a nameless innocent? This was what I had to prove, conclusively enough to satisfy police in Florida and New Hampshire.

There was a perplexing tab of bone from the male skeleton that seemed to float apart from the reconstruction, as it took shape. Composed of several fragments, dark gray and mottled in color, this flattened bone would provide me with a crucial, coinciding piece of evidence. It was the first, topmost rib of a male rib cage, short and stubby. Our ribs progress like harp strings, moving from small, short beginnings down to full, harmonious curves before shrinking again to the last, lowest ribs. This particular rib had a very irregularly shaped, calcified cartilage at the end nearest the breastbone. This nubbin of cartilage, this small irregularity, was extraordinarily distinctive. Under powerful illumination it stood out like a knot on a pine log.

A bright light and an old x-ray proved it was Meek's. In the early 1980s Meek had visited a chiropractor in Tucson, Arizona. I had not looked deeply into the dark areas of these x-rays, but now I used a special piece of equipment, a "hot spot," a bright reflecting bulb, to scrutinize the opaque and gloomy edges of these old x-rays. This powerful beam pierces the deepest shadows in x-ray films.

There, captured by the Arizona chiropractor and now illumined by the brilliant "hot spot," was the selfsame rib. The x-ray I took of the burned rib fragment, superimposed on the old chiropractor's x-ray, lined up magnificently. Exterior contours, interior irregularities, fell into place like a Euclidean theorem. The male rib from the fire belonged to Glyde Earl Meek. I did not fling up my arms or shout "Eureka!" but I will confess to experiencing a keen, silent elation while gazing at this eloquent bit of bone.

By now I had had a bellyful of New Hampshire state Attorney General Stephen Merrill's insinuations about the incompetence of Florida law enforcement officials and their dull-witted investigators. As late as June 1986, a year and a half after the murders, Merrill ostentatiously kept the case open and insisted on listing Meek as a living, wanted criminal. For this public and obstinate skepticism he won the huzzahs of the *Manchester Union Leader*.

> Merrill is to be commended for resisting the temptation to try to "close the book" on this sad, salacious controversy by accepting the facile conclusion that Page Jennings and Meek died in a fire in a High Springs, Florida shack on January 28th, 1985 [said an editorial in the *Union Leader* on June 4].
>
> It's not a question of the competence of the experts; it's a question of whether that competence is being extended beyond the area of their expertise. Merrill does not challenge the evidence. But, ever mindful of Meek's reputation as a devious convict, he notes that the teeth are not attached to bone, that in the past (in Arizona) Meek has saved his extracted teeth, and that there is a possibility of a "salting of the site" with phony evidence. . . .
>
> One can only wonder whether the Florida police, who have halted their search for Meek, are being equally precise in their consideration of the essential distinction between what the evidence indicates and what it proves. Merrill . . . deserves praise for demonstrating a high degree of professionalism in not accepting easy conclusions.

There were no such bouquets for me, toiling patiently in my little laboratory in Gainesville, poring over myriad flakes of reassembled bone. By now I was sure of my identifications, but I wished to "make assurance doubly sure." I determined to find the telltale gold filling that Meek had worn in life and was so conspicuously absent from his skeleton in death.

To do this I enlisted the services of three University of Florida archaeologists: Michael A. Russo, Charles R. Ewen and Rebecca Saunders. You can still examine our expense account in the files. We claimed for four pairs of leather gloves, ten dust masks and fifty Ziploc plastic bags. Using a tripod-mounted fine screen, with a

¹/₁₆-inch mesh, we excavated the complete shack down to sterile soil
—in vain. We did not find the gold inlay.

Then I directed that all the rocks, dirt and debris from the original spoil-piles—the material that had earlier been screened through
a ¹/₈-inch mesh—be brought back to the C. A. Pound Human Identification Laboratory and put through another, finer screen. This time
we would use a ¹/₁₆-inch mesh, about as fine as a window screen.

It was a young graduate student, Heidi Sydow, who found the
gold inlay. She was part of a work-study program and she more than
earned her pay that day. The crucial filling was caught at last, after
infinite pains and disappointments, sifted out in the fine mesh. A
single pin was bent, but the whole filling stood forth unmistakably.
Now it was captured in my hands, glittering with that imperishable
sparkle that has rendered gold so precious for thousands of years.
This fleck of gold, that day, was more precious to me than any other.

Pure gold melts at 1,945 degrees Fahrenheit. Dental gold is far
stronger. In a really hot structural fire, after eight hours of burning,
where the heat is most intense, it gets up to a little over 1,200
degrees Centigrade, or just under 2,300 degrees Fahrenheit. In my
experience I have seen aluminum and pot metals melt in house fires,
but seldom any metal more durable. To get to 1,945 degrees in a
house fire the blaze would have to continue as a raging fire for
around three hours. It is absurd to imagine the small shack in High
Springs burning for three hours at these terrific temperatures. The
galvanized tin roof sections that had collapsed into the fire were
unmelted. The Ithaca shotgun's slide was welded shut, but its barrel
was undeformed by the heat.

And in fact this gold filling had not melted either. Its original
shape was still clearly recognizable, and it was definitely Meek's. The
New Hampshire authorities clung feebly to their hypothesis—Meek
could have flung his gold filling into the fire! But soon after that Dr.
Mertz was able to prove that a whole fragment of the male jaw, with
teeth attached, corresponded to Meek's dental x-rays. Obviously he
had not flung his jaw into the fire.

After immense doubts and difficulties we had proved what

seemed likeliest at the very beginning of the case: Page Jennings and Glyde Earl Meek were dead. Their bones were the bones found in the burned cabin. The long and laborious investigation was closed. Glyde Earl Meek was finally, quietly taken off the "Most Wanted" list, and Stephen Merrill was elected governor of New Hampshire. His successor wrote me a friendly letter, apologizing for the doubts and difficulties stirred up over the Meek-Jennings affair. The most troublesome case I had ever encountered was finally solved.

Mixed with the sense of triumph was a bitter aftertaste of exasperation, because it took so much work to demonstrate beyond doubt what was from the very beginning the most probable solution. There was the feeling of having come round in a gigantic circle, after infinite and exhausting labor, to the simple starting point. "Reality," as Borges wrote, "has not the slightest obligation to be interesting. . . ."

But the long suicide note *was* interesting. What did its absurd, theatrical tale really mean? I have my own theories about its nuances.

I believe Glyde Earl Meek murdered Page Jennings shortly after she left her brother's apartment for the last time on January 11. I believe all the references to her joyous waiting, her deep meditations, her passive submission to strangulation, her loving acceptance of her death and cremation—all these are lies, made up by Meek to conceal the fact that he murdered a young girl and her parents because they dared to thwart him, stand in the path of his extravagant and all-encompassing dream of love and self-admiration. I believe he had every intention of murdering Chris Jennings too—the hatred for Chris fairly blazes from the suicide note, and the young man can count himself lucky he was not in his Gainesville apartment on January 18 when Meek came back from his homicidal errand in New Hampshire. I believe Meek entered the apartment bent on murder, using Page's key, only to find it unoccupied. Chris had gone to his parents' funeral in New Hampshire. That funeral saved his life.

184

What were Meek's thoughts as he traveled south from New Hampshire? Short on sleep, guilty of two, probably three, murders, nearly out of his mind, he may have toyed with the idea of substituting Chris Jennings's body for his own in the cabin. Meek had no idea how precise postmortem identifications of burned bones can be. He had already tried to hide the New Hampshire murders with a fire. Did he hope to cheat death and elude justice by placing Chris Jennings's body next to his dead sister's? "I would have taken all their lives anyway," he wrote in the note found in the meadow.

Enraged, exhausted and baffled to find Chris Jennings out of reach, Meek gave up, decided to die, and recrafted his suicide note to include an element of mercy. Chris Jennings, unexpectedly out of harm's way, would now be allowed to live after all, so that he could suffer endless pangs of remorse.

"You live with it all now, Bucko—Mal, Betty and us. Meddling fools," Meek wrote in the note left in Jennings's apartment. In the longer, more detailed note found in the Fiat he said:

> Her brother won't be harmed so that he can live with everything for the rest of his life. A pay back for rejecting her and writing that she was "insane" in his journal. Personally I would like to wait around and do him but she has made me promise not to give him the easy way out but to think about it every day. I have promised to go with her and so we shall.

Then, a few lines later in the same note:

> She is waiting now and I must do what I can't believe I'm going to do but I must do for me and her.

"Waiting" indeed! I believe Page Jennings was dead days before the fire in the cabin on January 18. Possibly her body was stored in the mini-warehouse during the hectic period between January 11 and January 18. The account of her strangulation rings true, but I believe it may very well have occurred long before her body was placed in the cabin to burn. I am still curious about the blood found on one of her Reebok sneakers. Where did it come from? When was it shed? Blood tests taken at the time revealed that the blood could have been Page Jennings's; DNA testing, the kind of testing we can do today, would leave absolutely no doubt. And I could wish, if that Reebok shoe were still available, that a careful DNA analysis might be run on that old blood smear. I believe the results would bear out my hypothesis, that Page was murdered, completely against her will.

To this day I feel pity for the bright young high school javelin thrower whose early life had been filled with such promise. That she would become the murdered child of murdered parents, that she would be strangled, brained and combusted to a heap of burned bones amid the ruins of a squalid, deserted shack a thousand miles from her home was an outcome as horrific as it was undeserved.

The buckshot in Meek's skull, as well as the lead traces on his lower jaw, make it clear that Meek used the shotgun on himself as the fire was kindled. If he used ropes to tie himself down, as he proclaimed in the suicide note, they were unnecessary. The shotgun blast killed him instantly.

Perhaps he hoped for some sort of fiery and final confusion, mingling his guilt with the innocence of the dead young woman beside him, his bones with hers. His final thoughts, as he pulled the trigger amid the licking flames, remain his alone. We possess only the leaden globules against the shattered and burned brainpan.

Chris Jennings left Gainesville, returned north and sold the inn his parents owned. He still sends me a Christmas card every year. It is a remembrance I appreciate.

Lost Legions

O stranger, go tell the Spartans
That here we lie, obedient to their orders.

—Simonides, 92D, *Epitaph for the 300 Spartans*
killed at Thermopylae

The question of American soldiers missing in action in Vietnam
is an open, bleeding wound in American politics even today. No
matter how many facts and reasonable arguments are sent into battle
against it, no matter how many congressional and military delega-
tions visit Hanoi, it seems this lingering ghost cannot be laid to rest.
The picture of gaunt, starved, tortured men housed in bamboo cages
in some trackless jungle has been reinforced in popular movies so
often now, that the existence of these poor wraiths has become an
article of faith for thousands of Americans. These soldiers were lost
in a lost war, and this twice-lost state has created an empty, gaping,
painful blank in America's soul.

Even though by now the term "MIA" has been superseded by
the more correct expression, "unaccounted for," nevertheless this
question has paralyzed American foreign policy toward Vietnam. It
still prevents full normalization of relations nearly two decades after

the cessation of hostilities. While only about 2200 men are still listed as unaccounted for from the Vietnam War, as opposed to 78,750 unaccounted for from World War II and 8,170 from the Korean War, it is the vanished soldiers of Vietnam who tug at our hearts and rob many of us of our reason today, long after the last guns have fallen silent.

Extraordinary legends have flourished over the years. There is said to be a warehouse somewhere in Hanoi, filled to the ceiling with the bones of U.S. servicemen, which are doled out one by one by the Vietnamese authorities in return for "concessions" on the part of the United States. There is a widespread and fantastic belief that the United States Government itself, to cover up its incompetence in failing to win the release of all American prisoners of war in 1973, has made an unholy alliance with Vietnam to hide the "truth" from the American public, i.e., that there are still Americans alive in prison camps in Southeast Asia, held hostage to Oriental malice.

MIAs have been honored on U.S. postage stamps; during the Reagan and Bush administrations, the black and white MIA flag flew once a year over the White House. It still flies today, on thousands of flagpoles across the country. There have even been video arcade games in which, for a succession of quarters, you could rescue these trapped Americans and be a hero. Confidence tricksters have preyed on survivors and their families, eliciting thousands of dollars in contributions, to pay for "reconnaissance and rescue missions," which somehow always fail by a hair's breadth to save any lost Americans.

When a delusion is as widely held and as firmly believed as the MIA scenario, it is perhaps futile to argue against it. I know nothing about this issue that is not already broad public knowledge. But I think if more Americans were aware of the immense concern and deep respect that is accorded to every single fragment of bone, no matter how tiny, that has been recovered in the search for these unaccounted-for men and women, then perhaps some of these widespread doubts and anxieties might be allayed.

I have firsthand knowledge of these efforts. Twice a year I visit the laboratory in Hawaii where recommendations for identifications are made and cases are resolved. I have seen and scrutinized the remains of our servicemen as they are brought home from Vietnam, in some cases after more than a quarter of a century. I have painstakingly double-checked many identifications myself, rejecting those I thought needed additional work. I continue to make recommendations to the Department of the Army for the improvement and enhancement of the identification process, and I can truthfully say that the military accepts most of my suggestions with a ready will and in a friendly spirit of cooperation.

The ceremony for receiving these honored dead in Hawaii is impressive. After a joint forensic review in Hanoi, Vietnamese officials return the remains in wooden boxes in Hanoi to their American counterparts. The wooden boxes are then placed in large aluminum cases that measure about six and a half feet long. The sides and tops of these cases are made from one piece of aluminum, which can be raised and lifted off the base. The cases are sealed, put aboard a transport plane in Hanoi, draped with American flags, and flown to Hickam Air Force Base, where they are met with full military honors.

In Hanoi it is usually U.S. army personnel, who carry the cases. In Hawaii they are carried off the planes by American servicemen in dress uniform from all of the branches of the service. In Hawaii the members of the honor guard march up the rear ramp of the C-141 Starlifter aircraft and carry off their dead comrades, one at a time. For ceremonial purposes, one aluminum case is treated as one body, even though within it there may be the commingled remains of several people. Hickam Field shares runway space with Honolulu International Airport and sometimes passengers on commercial flights get a glimpse of these solemn proceedings: the flags, the aluminum cases, the brass and braid of the honor guards twinkling against the green headlands of Hawaii and the wide, blue Pacific. They may not realize it, but they are witnessing one of the final chapters in our country's longest war.

I wish that those who suspect a vast conspiracy and cover-up could spend a few days inside the U. S. Army Central Identification

Laboratory (Hawaii), known by its acronym as CILHI. They would see one of the most modern, best-equipped forensic identification laboratories in the world. Within its walls some of the most searching and painstaking forensic identification work imaginable is carried out with every tool available to modern science.

The lab is a low structure that is not distinctive at all from the outside. It is a large affair, with more than 5,000 square feet of floor space. Inside a large, windowless, well-lit room are about twenty tables, each thirty inches wide by sixty inches long, arranged in rows. The remains on these tables are covered with sheets, and some are so pitifully small that they cause scarcely a ruffle in the clean white shroud. Every night as work ceases in the laboratory, the sheets are folded and arranged with military precision to cover the remains again. Signs at the door advise visitors that permission is required to enter, that no photographs are allowed and all headgear must be removed. This last injunction is strictly observed and is intended to show respect to the fallen.

At the end of the laboratory, in an L-shaped alcove, there are shelves built to hold the boxes of remains that have not been identified. There are *not* hundreds of such boxes, as some may imagine. At any given time the "unsolved" boxes number slightly over one hundred.

Microscopes are on worktables at one end of the room, and logbooks to enter receipts of the remains are near the front door. CILHI itself occupies only roughly half of this building. It is separated from the other half by a solid wall pierced by a single door that is always locked on both sides. The other half of the building is occupied by the military mortuary, which is intended to handle fresh remains. If there were some great disaster, such as a plane crash, both facilities would pitch in with their combined resources to process and identify the remains.

When the aluminum boxes are unsealed and the wooden boxes within are opened, the sight that greets the investigator is often anticlimactic. A miserably tiny scatter of small bones, so few you could hide them in your fist, may be all that is left of a supposed unaccounted-for serviceman. I say "supposed" advisedly. Though we believe the Vietnamese authorities are acting in good faith, it sometimes happens that the remains of one person may be scattered throughout several boxes. At the same time, portions of two crew mates may be commingled in one box. Often animal bones, or bones belonging to dead Vietnamese, may be present. The animal bones are carefully separated out. They are not thrown away but are usually kept in comparative collections, which are helpful in demonstrating what sort of animals may be found in the area where human remains turn up, and what to watch out for in future.

The Asiatic bones, which are classified as "Southeast Asian Mongoloid" in official terminology, are also winnowed out. These remains are sent back to Vietnam, although the authorities there are often unwilling to take them back. Soldiers who fought for the Republic of Vietnam—the south—during that long war are contemptuously known as *linh nguy* or "puppet soldiers" by the victorious North Vietnamese, and their graves are dishonored and overgrown by weeds. By contrast the North Vietnamese soldiers who died are called *bo doi phuc vien*, or "war veterans of the revolution," and their cemeteries are beautifully landscaped and festooned with flags every July 27 on Invalids and Fallen Heroes Day. Agreements formalized recently now permit American anthropologists to inspect the remains before accepting them for repatriation. This has greatly reduced the number of cases of mistaken racial identity.

This is how these remains are handled: Each new case is assigned to an anthropologist and, if there are any dental remains, to a forensic dentist as well. Obviously if the remains consist only of dental remains—one or several teeth—then there is nothing for an anthropologist to work on, and only a dentist would be called in. But in most instances you need both experts. Usually the anthropologist was present at the actual dig site, when the remains were unearthed.

The anthropologist and the dentist work independently of one another, so their conclusions can be cross-checked against each other. In most cases the dentist has a great advantage. He is usually privy to information, in the form of dental records, that the anthropologist does not have.

The dentist prepares a chart based on the dental evidence before him, and he is careful to show restorations, if the jaw has naturally missing teeth which fell out or were taken out while the subject was alive, and so on. After completing that descriptive phase, the dentist codes the information for entry into a computer. The computer, using software called Computer Assisted Post Mortem Identification (CAPMI), compares the entered information with the dental records stored in its data banks. More than 2500 dental records are in CAPMI. Now, that doesn't mean that the dental records of all 2200 unaccounted-for men are logged in CAPMI. Unfortunately, a few dozen lost soldiers have no dental records in the existing files today, and some men may have several files. The list of all unaccounted-for servicemen with dental records in CAPMI that are compatible with the unknown remains appears on the screen and can be printed out.

To give an example: if all that is present is an upper right first molar, which is tooth No. 3 in the universal system, and this tooth has an amalgam restoration in the occlusal or biting surface, this is entered into CAPMI in abbreviated code: "Tooth No. 3 has an O-AM," or an occlusal amalgam restoration. Every individual record in CAPMI with an O-AM would immediately pop up on the computer screen. But the program doesn't quit there. It lists every individual who had *no* restorations in No. 3, according to their latest dental records. Why? Because there is always a possibility that a filling was added later and was not recorded.

However, a person with a No. 3 with a restoration in the occlusal surface *and another restoration in the lingual surface* of the tooth would be *excluded* by the program and not listed. As we say: "Teeth don't heal." In short, people with a tooth with *too few* restorations could still be considered; but a tooth with *too many* would be ruled out by CAPMI.

Obviously in this example the list of possibilities would be very long indeed. But if more teeth are present, with more variables, the list shortens considerably. In any case the dentist must go to the actual dental x-rays and compare them to the postmortem dental x-rays. This may be very time-consuming work requiring great patience. If a radiographic match cannot be made, other information is factored in. Where were the remains recovered? Where were the individuals lost? If the plane crash is known from our records, if our team excavated the site in cooperation with a team from the former belligerent country, then we concentrate the initial search on those crew members involved in that incident whose names appear in CAPMI.

Let us leave the dentist for the moment. While he is working with names and records, the anthropologist, who has only the bones before him, is wholly in the dark as to the possible identification. This is done deliberately, to prevent any preconceptions or foregone conclusions. He or she must reach conclusions based on the number of individuals represented, which bones go with which individual, the age, sex, race, height and so forth of each individual lying before him. It would be so rare as to be almost miraculous that an anthropologist would develop information that itself would lead to the identification of a particular serviceman. But the anthropologist's independence from the dentist later becomes vitally important when a dental identification is made. The anthropologist's findings are extremely important when the process of cross-checking begins, in order to establish that the skeletal remains are consistent with the dental identification.

Obviously all this painstaking work is not accomplished over a few days' time. Indeed, the anthropologist may be interrupted and have to set the case aside, to return to Southeast Asia for another recovery effort. But little by little each set of remains is thoroughly examined. In the end, the laboratory director receives a full report. There is the dental summary from the dentist. There is the anthropological summary from the anthropologist. There is the incident information, including maps of locations and other material brought forth from the records room. There is the search and recovery report from the search and recovery team. Finally, there is the death certificate, signed by an army pathologist at Tripler Army Medical Center after reviewing the findings of the case.

The laboratory director forwards the combined file, with his recommendation for identification, to the laboratory commander, an army colonel, who then forwards it to Washington. The office in Washington sends complete duplicates of these case files, including photographs and x-rays, to me. Nor am I the sole recipient. There is a pool of forensic anthropologists and forensic dentists currently under contract to the Army to double-check these lab findings. All of us are board-certified by our respective disciplines, and we are considered to have reached a certain degree of prominence in our fields, so that our opinions carry the weight of reputation. I've been under contract to the Army since 1986 and have flown to CILHI in Hawaii many times since then; and I have examined findings in my laboratory here in Gainesville oftener still. In fact I was involved in the discussions that led to the setting up of this process. Over the years nine people have had contracts at one time or another to provide this consulting service.

After I (or another of my colleagues under contract) have meticulously reviewed the file, we have the option of either flagging it or approving it. If we flag it, the case will be put on hold until we have an opportunity to examine the remains ourselves. We may also recommend that more work be done or additional documents be prepared. But the standards at CILHI are very high now, and in most cases the reviewer finds that the identification is scientifically valid. He then returns the dossier, together with his written review, to Washington. This is what happens in most cases.

Now comes the moment when the family is finally notified. The branch of service in which the man served sends its mortuary affairs officer, who is a funeral director, to visit the family and explain the findings and the reviews. At that time the family has the option of accepting the findings, or, if they so choose, having their own expert examine the remains and review the file. This almost never happens and, on those rare occasions when it has, the outside expert has

never succeeded in finding evidence that would overthrow the recommended identification.

But even now the process isn't quite finished. With the family's
concurrence, the files, with all of the reviews, including that of the
family's consultant (if they decided to hire one), goes to the Armed
Forces Identification Review Board (AFIRB). AFIRB consists of
officers in the various branches of service who hold the rank of 0–6
(that is, a colonel in the Army or Air Force, a captain in the Navy).
Most of these officers have served in Southeast Asia under the same
conditions as the men who were lost. They understand from their
own experience what conditions were then, and are now, in that
theater of war. If they agree with the recommendation, it then goes
to the Graves Registration Office, for final approval.

The remains, which have stayed in the Hawaii laboratory all this
time, are taken in flag-covered transfer cases from CILHI to the
adjacent Hickam Field, where they are loaded onto military aircraft
by an honor guard of the branch in which they served. They are then
flown to a mortuary in the continental United States where they are
placed in a casket with full uniform and appropriate decorations and
insignia. The remains then go to the national cemetery or to a home-
town cemetery, just as the next of kin wish.

We cannot work miracles, however. It is a fact that some remains
stay in the L-shaped room adjacent to the laboratory for years, and a
handful may never be identified. Every year additional records are
sifted for comparison. There is always the hope that additional portions of remains will come in, or that some clue will jog an investigator's memory, leading to a file on an unaccounted-for serviceman
that turns out to be the correct one. But in these stubborn, residual
cases, where the dental and skeletal evidence is sparse, the investigators face a formidable task. Some of these bones literally come from
nowhere; we do not even have the name of the spot within Vietnam,
Laos or Cambodia where they were unearthed. That information has
been lost. Yet the bones are retained, year after year, and are often
taken down and studied afresh, over and over again.

———

The task of identifying unaccounted-for remains at CILHI is immense and never ending. Alas, honesty compels me to admit that the laboratory did not always function as smoothly and professionally as it does today. As a congressional inquiry later revealed, some identifications made at CILHI were based on conclusions that were only inadequately backed up by evidence. I discovered this for myself when I visited CILHI as an outside expert in 1985. My involvement with the laboratory stemmed from a plane crash over Laos many years earlier, and from the persistence of one devoted widow who could not forget the loss of her husband.

Four days before Christmas, on December 21, 1972, an AC-130A gunship was shot down over Laos near a place called Pakse. The AC-130A was on a mission to attack North Vietnamese vehicles moving south along the Ho Chi Minh trail, which at that point wandered through supposedly neutral Laotian territory. The AC-130A is a formidable gunship, a modified Lockheed Hercules C-130 transport plane, which is still very much a part of America's aerial armory. It has seen service in Somalia recently. Stuffed with computers and radar, carrying a crew normally numbering fifteen, bristling with cannons and machine guns with electronic firing pins, which blast bullets downward in a well-nigh solid stream of murderous metal, the craft is a slow-flying dreadnaught capable of immense, accurate destruction.

But on this day the plane was hit by antiaircraft fire from below and fuel began to flow into the fuselage, soaking the crew and the huge stores of ammunition aboard. A survivor later spoke of wading through this highly flammable fuel as it sloshed about inside the doomed aircraft. The pilot desperately steered his stricken plane toward Thailand and safety, but soon realized the situation was hopeless. Remaining at the controls, he gallantly ordered the other crew members to head for the rear, open ramp of the Hercules. That day there were sixteen men aboard the aircraft; the plane was carrying one extra crewman.

The other crew members were on their way aft, ready to parachute to safety, when the plane gave a jolt and spun out of control.

In one cataclysmic second the fuel ignited and exploded. Two men were blown out of the rear of the craft and parachuted safely to the jungle below. There they were picked up and rescued by search and rescue aircraft and taken to safety in neighboring Thailand. They were the only survivors. It is believed that the other fourteen men, including the navigator, Lieutenant Colonel Thomas Trammell Hart III, perished when the AC-130A plunged into the jungle at a high angle of impact and burned, its cargo of thousands of rounds of ammunition exploding in the fire.

A day or so later a human arm was found in the jungle by some local friendly forces and was returned to U.S. military personnel, where it was identified by fingerprints as one of the members of the crew. His body was thus accounted for at that time. The rest of the crew members were officially listed as "missing in action."

In 1985, I received a telephone call from Lieutenant Colonel Hart's widow. She told me that she was active in the League of Families, a support organization trying to resolve cases of relatives missing in action. Not content with the official account of the crash, this resolute, plucky woman had visited the crash site in Laos and gone over the ground herself. Not only that: she had actually picked up bone fragments from the surface and turned them over to American authorities. She told me that later a CILHI group had worked jointly with a team from Laos to excavate the crash site and recover the remains of the dead personnel, but she confided that she had no faith whatever in the CILHI laboratory or its personnel. At this point CILHI had not yet made any identifications of the Pakse remains, but even so Mrs. Hart was skeptical. She was not prepared to accept CILHI's word when it came to her husband's remains. She wanted independent confirmation. My name had been mentioned to her by a colleague in Colorado, Dr. Michael Charney, and she asked me for a second opinion. She wanted me to examine personally the remains said to be those of her husband.

I said I would. She asked how much I would charge. I said I would not charge anything to assist the family of a lost serviceman. Unfortunately, I had to go to China that summer to give a series of lectures on the identification of air crash victims. When I returned, I found out that CILHI had indeed identified one set of remains as Lieutenant Colonel Hart's. Since I was unavailable, Mrs. Hart had gone to Dr. Charney, who performed the second examination.

Charney made no secret of his disagreement with the official army identification of Lieutenant Colonel Hart's remains. In interviews given to the news media he accused CILHI of practicing "voodoo science" to identify these remains. The Pakse case received such wide attention that in December 1985 I received another telephone call, this time from one of the most distinguished figures in forensic anthropology, Dr. Ellis Kerley, a professor at the University of Maryland, whose reputation was legendary.

Kerley asked me if I would be interested in joining a three-man commission of anthropologists, which the United States Army had asked him to form, to visit and evaluate CILHI. I agreed but advised Kerley that, instead of having a third anthropologist, what we really needed was a forensic dentist. Teeth can be crucial in identifying human remains. Kerley then invited Dr. Lowell Levine, an internationally known forensic dentist from New York, and we all received invitational travel orders from the Army to visit the laboratory. Ellis was to write an unclassified written summary of our findings. And so we flew to Hawaii.

Science can be a cruel discipline sometimes, and the truth can cut deeply. Ellis Kerley found himself in a terrible position soon after arriving in Hawaii and entering the CILHI laboratory. He was being called upon to evaluate the work of one of his oldest friends, Tadao Furue, an honest and upright Japanese scientist with a remarkable history. Furue had been chosen as a kamikaze pilot in the closing days of World War II and only the quick end of the war after the United States dropped atomic bombs on Hiroshima and Nagasaki had prevented him from climbing into his plane and immolating himself as a human bomb for his Emperor.

After the war Furue went to college in Tokyo and, while yet a student, was hired by a U.S. military laboratory in Japan to assist in the identification of American soldiers killed in combat. Some of the greatest names in forensic anthropology were active in this work, including my teacher, Tom McKern, as well as Mildred Trotter, the famous anatomist and human osteologist, and T. Dale Stewart, the curator of physical anthropology at the Smithsonian Museum of Natural History, who had for years performed the analyses of human remains for the FBI and other governmental agencies. Kerley, too, had worked at the Tokyo laboratory during the Korean War. En route to Japan, aboard ship, Kerley met his future wife, Mary, who was traveling with the USO. When they were married in Japan, Tadao Furue had been Ellis's best man.

Furue remained in Japan after the U. S. Army lab closed. From time to time his services were used by other mortuaries, whenever he was needed. In those days there was no central identification laboratory. In the early years of the Vietnam War all the identifications of dead U.S. soldiers were carried out in individual military mortuaries. It was only as the war wound down that a central identification laboratory was opened in Thailand. When that laboratory relocated in the 1970s to Honolulu, Furue was employed for the first time away from Japan as the anthropologist.

Now Ellis Kerley found himself in the delicate position of passing judgment on the work of the man who had stood up for him at his wedding. Ellis found the situation excruciating. He is one of the most gentle men you could ever hope to meet. I can picture him saying to a student who flubbed an examination: "Well, Mr. Smith, you *really* didn't do as well as you *might* have on this examination and we are going to have to *ask* you to take the course over again." He would never be so brutal as to say: "You flunked." Ellis is the soul of discretion, a man who would bend over backward to spare people's feelings.

The laboratory, when we visited it in 1985, was made up of two buildings. There was the administration building, a two-story cinderblock affair; and a one-story warehouse-like building next door, made of a corrugated material, probably asbestos, with a nicely finished interior. Furue had a large office in one corner that was separated from the laboratory floor by the x-ray room, whose unshielded walls housed the dental x-ray machine. This machine was the only radiographic facility in the laboratory.

All of the anthropological instruments in the laboratory were Furue's. The entire reference library—mostly books in Japanese— belonged to him. The laboratory's array of photographic equipment was so limited that, when Furue wanted to document specimens, he used his own camera, bought his own film and often had the film processed at his own expense. The pictures in the laboratory files therefore didn't even legally belong to the government. They were Furue's own personal property. There wasn't even a hot-water heater in the building.

One end of the laboratory was divided off into a records room where all the medical records on the unaccounted for were housed. Also available there were condensed mortuary records on every serviceman and woman who had been killed in Southeast Asia and identified at the mortuaries that preceded CILHI.

We had only two and a half days in the laboratory so we had to work quickly. We naturally focused on the Pakse case as a kind of convenient benchmark, a recent example of the laboratory's methods. This was, after all, the case that had aroused official concern because of the inquiries by Lieutenant Colonel Hart's widow. As the hours passed and the three of us sat around the table looking at files and notebooks, a feeling of dread gradually took hold and spread among us. We were being pushed inexorably toward a painful conclusion: some of Furue's identifications of the Pakse remains simply would not hold water.

At the beginning of the summer of 1985, CILHI had announced that every single one of the thirteen lost men had been identified from the bone and dental fragments gathered on site in Laos. All these remains would be returned to their families. The whole crew had been accounted for. Furue told us with pride that approximately 50,000 bone and tooth fragments had been recovered from the crash site. Those, along with the fragments Mrs. Hart had collected, had been analyzed by him with the help of his assistants. They had separated out all the fragments that might be used for identification. As we looked at his photographs, we began to see that many of the identifications were made on distressingly little evidence indeed, based on an examination of the scantiest of remains. Even when more complete skeletal remains were available, there were still some grave difficulties.

Tadao and his assistant had tried to separate out the Pakse remains into neat piles, by age and size. Unfortunately in this case all of the crew members were white, all of them were male, and most of them were young. They ranged in age from nineteen to forty-one. In some cases, teeth were missing from the sets of remains altogether. The sum total of one set of remains was a single fragment of the shoulder area. Any identification based on such meager remains, with no additional evidence such as DNA test results, is bound to be mere wishful thinking.

We said in our report that in only five of the Pakse cases could identifications be substantiated from dental evidence. This was a far cry from the thirteen positive identifications Furue and his assistants had announced.

Tadao is dead now, so I can speak of him without wounding his pride; for he was a man of intense pride, who set himself the impossible goal of accounting for every single one of the lost servicemen in Vietnam if at all possible. The phrase, "fullest possible accounting," which is so often heard from opponents of normalizing relations with Vietnam, and which is an utter impossibility, became for Tadao Furue a real goal to be aimed at. Ultimately this unreachable standard of perfection led to his downfall. He became so obsessed with the identification process that he would reach conclusions in cases where no answer was possible. He was a perfect gentleman, rigorously moral in his personal life, one of the courtliest men I've ever met, but I think he suffered from the intellectual isolation of being alone in the laboratory. The very confidential nature of the military identification process itself inhibits free discussion. Unable to confer with students and colleagues in the field, working practically alone in a laboratory thousands of miles from the U.S. mainland, Tadao was literally and intellectually cut off.

It became our painful duty to inform the Defense Department that the CILHI laboratory needed a serious overhaul. The three of us returned home and drew up our reports. Ellis, instead of preparing the final report himself, submitted our three reports separately and independently. My report was probably the most critical of the three and, since these documents were not classified, they created quite a stir when they were released to the media in January 1986. ABC's "20-20" news journal put together a segment on the CILHI laboratory and this created an unpleasant ruckus in the Defense Department. Blaming the bearer of bad tidings is only human nature. Everyone who has been in uniform knows how unpleasantness tends to roll downhill in the armed forces.

Our immediate reward for being so frank about CILHI was to be subjected to a loud, private harangue by a member of the White House's national security advisers—an officer who was one of Lieutenant Colonel Oliver North's associates, and whose name I have no wish to recall. This unforgettable, high-decibel tirade occurred well after I thought the whole CILHI affair had been laid to rest. It lasted four weary hours one evening and took place in the Executive Office Building next door to the White House, in a room adjacent to that in which the Iran Contra papers were so assiduously shredded to long confetti. The officer loudly protested our findings. We had opened a Pandora's box of endless mischief! I was accused of ruining Tadao's life, of having robbed him of the will to live, even of causing the liver cancer from which he now suffered! I have seen many disturbing sights in the autopsy room, but the spectacle of this enraged colonel, sitting a few hundred yards from the very pinnacle of power, disturbed me more deeply than many a ghastly corpse. Were such illogical men really in charge of our national security? I emerged shaken and angry from this ordeal.

Happily the angry colonel's views were not shared by others in the military. In early 1986, I was invited to testify at a hearing of the Veterans Affairs Committee at the U. S. Senate. After my testimony I was invited by Major General John Crosby, who had also testified on behalf of the Army, to join him for lunch at the Pentagon. Crosby was an extraordinary officer, a man who radiated an air of command and brisk efficiency. I told him frankly that I believed any problems within CILHI could be corrected if we all worked together, instead of at cross-purposes. General Crosby agreed with me and over the months that followed we were gratified to see nearly all the reforms we had proposed carried out at CILHI.

Toward the end of 1986, General Crosby invited us back to the laboratory for a follow-up visit. Soon the three of us found ourselves under contract to review all identifications recommended by the laboratory involving Southeast Asian casualties. This review process continues to this day. Ellis Kerley became chief of the laboratory for several years but is now retired and living in Hawaii. Today CILHI has several civilian consultants. Lowell and I are the most active, but there are others who watch over the laboratory on a less frequent basis. Tadao Furue was handled gently. He was kept on as senior anthropologist at the facility, but his role became more and more an advisory one. He died a few years later.

Now I visit CILHI twice a year. Besides reviewing every single case recommended for identification, my colleagues and I discuss CILHI's personnel needs, its staff, improvements in equipment and such stuff. Often we huddle over a set of remains and make suggestions as to what more might be done to identify them. At other times we play devil's advocates, challenging age estimates and other conclusions. Fresh air and free debate make every identification more reliable and trustworthy.

The search for unaccounted-for servicemen does not stop at CILHI's laboratory doors. Year in and year out, you will find teams from CILHI in the field, actively searching for and recovering the remains of our lost soldiers. In the rain forests of New Guinea they can be found investigating the hundreds of plane crashes left over from World War II. In the mountains and gorges of South Korea they are busy seeking out the dead from some long-forgotten battle, reclaiming them from the shallow graves where they were buried by returning villagers. There is a full-time American-run search office near Hanoi. Expeditions still comb Vietnam, north and south, as well as Laos and Cambodia. Here the anthropologists and the army investigators alike wear civilian clothes, as the Vietnamese do not permit American uniforms to be worn in the countryside. Their work can be dangerous. Some of the personnel in the laboratory wear Purple Hearts for wounds received many years ago in such search-and-recover missions. Recently one CILHI team in Cambodia came under fire from Khmer Rouge guerrillas. Lately the North Koreans have been turning over sets of U.S. servicemen's remains from that more than forty-year-old conflict, and these too, must be identified.

Unfortunately, the Pakse case ended messily. Doubts over the unidentified remains persisted and in 1986, after I had done my report on CILHI but before I signed a contract with the Army to conduct an ongoing review of the lab, I was asked by Mrs. Hart to look again at the remains of her husband. I agreed.

The remains were brought to my laboratory in Gainesville in a full-sized casket with a military escort. The lid of the great polished casket was opened—to disclose seven tiny bits of bone. I thoroughly described each fragment and what conclusions could be drawn in terms of age, weight, height and so on. The Army then asked Ellis Kerley to review the Hart case, as well as the independent reports made by Dr. Charney in Colorado and myself in Florida. Based on this evidence, Ellis recommended that the identification of Lieutenant Colonel Hart be rescinded. Later another identification from Pakse was rescinded as well.

Concerning this pair of rescinded identifications, an important point must be made: the fact that the identifications were rescinded means that the available evidence, on which the identifications had been made, was later found to be inadequately proven in the collective opinion of the reviewing scientists. In other words, the evidence in these two cases did not meet reasonable levels of scientific certainty. But I want it understood clearly that there were no findings of *misidentifications* in these disputed cases, and there is absolutely no evidence to support any such charge.

Mrs. Hart sued the government and won approximately

$500,000; but the government appealed and ultimately won its case. The persistent widow, whose honest doubts had led to a thorough reform of CILHI, was not able to prove in court that CILHI's over-confident identification of her husband, even though it was based on such limited evidence, was "intentional and malicious," as she had claimed in her lawsuit. Another family, whose son was also identified after Pakse, was so incensed that they scorned to accept his alleged remains, giving them instead to Dr. Charney, who uses them as a lecture exhibit to demonstrate evidence used to make some military identifications.

This bitter aftermath vividly shows how painful and vexatious the whole question is, how different is the emotional response of each family it touches. Some want to get the whole thing behind them, and some will never sleep until they have vengeance. I make it a point to avoid contact with the families. Their emotions would cloud my objectivity; and frankly, I do not want to tell them the terrible tales of violence and suffering told me by those bones. I will say no more here, beyond what most people already know: that death in combat is not always quick, clean or painless, and the remains of our soldiers are sometimes maltreated after death, as we have all seen on television as recently as October 1993, in the streets of Mogadishu, in Somalia.

During my first visit to CILHI—which, for all I knew then, would be my last—I took a few minutes out to attend to some personal business. My wife had a roommate in college whose brother had been a pilot in Vietnam. His jet had crashed, and he had been killed; but his body had been recovered. Taking advantage of my unique access to the laboratory, I asked to see the young man's mortuary records just before I left. To my relief, I found that the young pilot had been identified by dental records as well as by fingerprints. As I closed the records I knew that, if my wife's college roommate ever asked me this awful question, I could reassure her that there was absolutely no mistake about her brother's identification.

What does the future hold for CILHI and the whole process of identifying our unaccounted-for war dead? As time goes on, the recovered bone fragments are growing smaller and smaller, the teeth scarcer and scarcer. As a result, identifications are obviously getting harder and harder to make. It is not hard to foresee a day, not very long distant, when CILHI will have to rely on DNA analysis to identify these remains, rather than go through the grindingly slow process of physically examining minuscule bits of skeletal material. By comparing DNA samples recovered from the remains with that of living relatives, identities could be established beyond all reasonable doubt, in weeks rather than years.

I must hasten to add that CILHI doesn't have the capability to do such DNA matching right now, at least not on the grand scale needed to close out the Vietnam files, let alone the even older and more fragmentary remains that are coming in from South and North Korea. Such a task lies beyond the combined capacity of all the DNA laboratories in the United States, at present. I should therefore like to see CILHI establish its own DNA lab, devoted exclusively to its own casework on our unaccounted-for servicemen. It would not be cheap. But the sum would be small indeed, compared to the mountains of money spent waging the Vietnam War.

I have seen the names of the Pakse crew on the famous Vietnam memorial wall in Washington. For me, as for most visitors, the wall is a deeply moving experience. But I am touched almost as deeply when I visit Arlington National Cemetery and see the grave of the Unknown Soldier from Vietnam. To the end of his life, my friend Tadao Furue lamented that these remains had been wrested prematurely from his care, taken from CILHI and buried in Washington.

I remember Tadao shaking his head in frustration and telling me: "If they had only given me more time! I could have identified him!" Tadao's spirit was unconquerable. Could he have made this Unknown Soldier known? One can only wonder. Heavy slabs of marble now guard the nameless warrior forever.

13

The Misplaced Conquistador

At length, Pizarro, unable, in the hurry of the moment, to adjust the fastenings of his cuirass, threw it away, and, enveloping one arm in his cloak, with the other seized his sword, and sprang to his brother's assistance. It was too late; for Alcantara was already staggering under the loss of blood and soon fell to the ground. Pizarro threw himself on his invaders, like a lion roused in his lair, and dealt his blows with as much rapidity and force, as if age had no power to stiffen his limbs. "What ho!" he cried, "Traitors! have you come to kill me in my own house?"

— William H. Prescott, *History of the Conquest of Peru*,
    Book 4, Chap. 5

Francisco Pizarro died as he lived, by the sword. When the rapiers of his assassins pricked his gullet, they extinguished a life that was all strife and struggle. Illegitimate and illiterate, a foundling in infancy and a swineherd in youth, he made his way to South America and, by pure force of will, toppled one of the greatest empires the world has seen. He enriched himself, his family and the King of Spain beyond the dreams of avarice. Indomitable in adversity, ruthless in victory, Pizarro and his followers laid waste utterly to the Inca

civilization whose ruined monuments dazzle us still; whose Cyclo-
pean walls, golden masks and inscrutable pictographs are so extraordinary they almost seem not of this earth. But when it came to
sharing out this almost immeasurable loot, Pizarro and his associates
became embroiled in blood feuds that proved fatal. At the very
height of his powers, the warlord of conquered Peru was assassinated.

Thanks to the faithful chroniclers of New Spain, we know nearly
as much about Pizarro's assassination in 1541 as we do about many
political murders in our own century. Because of the extraordinary
continuity of Spanish civilization in the conquered continent, we can
follow the story of his bones almost year by year.

I have held this old sinner's skull in my hands. The trauma marks
still visible on Pizarro's remains bear astonishing witness to the terrible fury of his attackers. Modern assassins have the tremendous
explosive force of firearms at their disposal. Pizarro's slayers wielded
swords alone; but what sword steel could do to the human skull and
skeletal frame it did to Francisco Pizarro. He died brutally and painfully, as the multiple nicks and scorings of his bones attest. His
skeleton can stand comparison with several modern murder victims
I have examined, for the atrocity of the wounds it reveals.

There is a powerful magic in the past. When we touch a human
artifact from centuries or millennia ago, we seem to behold our
brother human beings from across the deeps of time. If we are not
careful, we fall into dreams of bygone days and the light of sunsets
long extinguished. I have seen cool, analytical, clear-brained colleagues, especially my archaeologist friends, practically swooning
with admiration over some small potsherd, all but overcome by the
mere physical presence of human antiquity. "Just think!" they will
say in hushed voices. "This is the very such-and-such that once belonged to so-and-so!"

I envy them this second sight, this gift of imaginative reverie; but
I cannot afford to share the mood. I have been called to far countries
to examine remains of considerable age, and have handled things
vested with exceptional historical significance, but I can't permit

myself the luxury of time travel on these occasions. The clock is ticking. Work has to be done. Accuracy is all. As Margaret Thatcher admonished George Bush in the emergency days after Iraq invaded Kuwait: "Now, George, this is no time to go wobbly!" On such occasions I am more likely to worry about electric voltage and adapters, whether our equipment will work, whether we have brought enough film and instruments, whether we have sufficient spare parts if something breaks. I cannot spare time to muse about vanished greatness and departed glory. I cannot afford to go wobbly.

Yet when I look back on the case of the misplaced conquistador, Francisco Pizarro, I am struck by how neatly the pieces fell into position, and how the remains dovetailed exactly with historical accounts of the man. Pizarro's were the first really famous bones I handled, and the investigation into his death marked my first foray into historical forensic anthropology. Together with several colleagues, I was able to unmask an impostor mummy, which for years had been displayed and reverenced as the body of the conquistador. At the same time, I was able to help authenticate another set of skeletal remains as belonging beyond any doubt to the man who conquered Peru for Spain. A careful reconstruction of facial features, built up from the true skull, has given us a reasonable portrait of what Pizarro looked like in life. The verified bones have been put in their rightful place of honor in Lima's Cathedral of San Agustín, and a case of mistaken identity has been solved for good.

There was a time when every schoolchild knew of the astonishing exploits of Francisco Pizarro, the self-made soldier of fortune from Trujillo, Spain, who went to Panama with Vasco Nuñez de Balboa, the first European discoverer of the Pacific Ocean. At the age of fifty, an old man by the reckoning of his time, Pizarro embarked on the conquest of Peru. This climaxed in 1532 with his famous march to Cajamarca, deep in the Peruvian interior, with sixty-seven horses and a mere hundred and ten soldiers, not more than twenty of whom were armed, and these only with crossbows or arquebuses. Atahualpa, the Inca King, was waiting for him there with an army of 40,000 to 50,000 men, but was strangely paralyzed by indecision. Atahualpa allowed Pizarro to take possession of the citadel of Cajamarca and camped with his Inca army on the plains below. Invited to a parley, the Inca chief entered the citadel with only a few hundred followers. There he was ambushed and captured by Pizarro's men, who slaughtered the King's courtiers and raped his concubines. Overnight, almost at a stroke, the empire of the Incas was laid low, its King taken prisoner.

Then comes the famous tale of the Room of Gold. In return for his life and freedom, Atahualpa offered to fill with gold a room twenty-two feet long and seventeen feet wide to a height of seven feet. Pizarro agreed but also demanded that an adjacent room, somewhat smaller, be filled twice over with silver.

Five months later the larger room was still not quite full, even though a total of 1,326,539 gold pesos had been amassed. One fifth of the treasure was sent back to Spain and the remainder was divided among Pizarro and his men. Once the gold was disposed of, Atahualpa had no further value to Pizarro. To get rid of him, Pizarro had the Inca tried on trumped-up charges of insurrection, embezzling funds, adultery and idol-worshiping. He was found guilty and, two hours after sundown on July 16, 1533, was led to the stake to be burned. Atahualpa only avoided this atrocious mode of execution by "converting" to Christianity at the stake, and being baptized as "Juan de Atahualpa." Pizarro then had the Inca chief garroted.

The Spaniards proceeded to tear the Inca Empire to shreds and divide its spoils. A puppet king installed by Pizarro, Toparca, died mysteriously. Atahualpa's bravest general, Challcuchima, was burned at the stake. The last Inca army, led by a general named Quizquiz, was destroyed utterly by Pizarro's bitter rival, an old, one-eyed veteran named Diego de Almagro. On November 15, 1533, the Inca capital, Cuzco, fell. With it came more than half a million pesos' worth of gold. The victorious conquistadors rampaged across the land, using the Incas' own highways to travel, all the while slaughtering flocks, confiscating crops, despoiling temples and causing farmland and irrigation systems to fall into ruin. The unrestrained cruelty of the conquest of Peru still arouses our horror and pity.

Deprived of most of the booty by Pizarro and his brothers, Almagro and his men were understandably outraged. Pizarro offered Almagro the country of Chile, and the old soldier marched off, hoping to duplicate Pizarro's success. But Chile held no gold to compare with the riches of Peru. Almagro and his men endured two years of terrible war and physical hardship, emerging from Chile empty-handed and furious with Pizarro and his brothers, who were now in possession of all the Inca wealth. After a series of battles and double crosses, Almagro was defeated at Las Salinas on April 26, 1538, captured and executed by the garrote, on the orders of Pizarro's brother, Hernando. Pizarro himself later stripped Almagro's son of his lands, leaving the young man and his followers penniless and desperate for revenge. Pizarro was now governor of Peru, ruling from Lima, which he had founded in 1535.

The younger Almagro and his supporters spun a plot to kill Pizarro at mass on Sunday, June 26, 1541. One of the conspirators whispered of the plot while confessing his sins to a priest, who broke the sacred and confidential seal of confession and informed Pizarro of the danger. Pizarro seems to have shrugged off the warning but, as a precaution, feigned illness and did not attend mass that Sunday. He shared the story with the vice-mayor, Juan Belásquez, who assured the governor that he was safe as long as the "rod of justice" was in Belásquez's hands. With these assurances, Pizarro sat down to his Sunday dinner with about twenty guests seated around the table, including his half brother, Francisco Martín de Alcántara, Belásquez and other cavaliers.

It was the last meal he would ever eat. While he was yet at table, a tumult was heard outside the governor's palace. The conspirators charged across the Plaza de Armas outside the governor's mansion, shouting their intentions. There is confusion about their number: some accounts say there were as few as seven, some as many as twenty-five. Pizarro kept his head and calmly ordered the front door of the palace to be locked. The officer sent to do this, Francisco Hurtado de Hevia, unwisely chose to negotiate with the aggressors through the half-open door. They forced their way in with a great clamor. Hearing this uproar, most of Pizarro's dinner guests promptly deserted him, among them Belásquez, who climbed down into the garden with his "rod of justice" firmly grasped in his mouth.

Now began Pizarro's last battle. The old conquistador attempted to buckle on his armor breastplate, but the bulky leather straps would not fasten in time. Dropping the armor and wrapping a cloak around his left arm for a shield, he rushed to meet his assailants, who were already fighting with Alcántara and three or four loyal men.

Because several of the conspirators survived to be interrogated under torture, we know more or less what happened next, blow by blow. By the time Pizarro joined the fray, most of his defenders were dead or dying, including Alcántara. Finding himself alone, the doughty old warrior taunted his opponents and killed at least two of them. After he ran his sword into a third, a man standing behind this conspirator shoved the transfixed body forward, impaling the dying man further on Pizarro's weapon. While Pizarro was wrestling with the blade, trying to pull it free, he received a rapier wound in his throat, which disabled him. Falling to the floor, bleeding, he was swiftly surrounded by the remaining conspirators, who plunged their blades into him. He may have been shot with a crossbow bolt as well. According to one account, he asked for water as he lay dying, and a soldier named Barragan broke a water jug over his head, telling him he could have his next drink in hell.

"He fought so long with them that with very weariness, his sword fell out of his hands, and then they slew him with a prick of a rapier through his throat: and when he was fallen to the ground, and his wind failing him, he cried unto God for mercy, and when he had so done, he made a cross on the ground and kissed it, and then incontinent yielded up the ghost," wrote a contemporary historian, Garcilaso de la Vega in his *Royal Commentaries*.

Like the assassins who murdered Julius Caesar centuries before, the victorious conspirators all dipped their swords in Pizarro's blood, to share in the honor of the deed. Some discussed cutting Pizarro's head off, but this was finally vetoed. A near riot broke out in Lima because of the murder, which the clergy attempted to quell by parading the holy eucharist in procession around the city. That night Doña Inés Muñoz, the wife of Alcántara, buried the body of her husband, together with that of Pizarro, behind the cathedral on the side facing the Plaza de Armas.

But Pizarro's remains were not destined to rest in peace. Four years after his death, in 1545, came the first of many reburials and relocations: the conqueror's bones and swords were exhumed and deposited in a wooden box under the main altar of the Lima cathedral, according to a wish expressed in his will. In 1551, Doña Francisco Pizarro Yupanqui, the daughter of the conquistador, and Doña Inés Yupanqui Huaylas, another relative, gave five thousand measures of gold to construct a special chapel in the cathedral for Pizarro's remains. Money was also donated to assure perpetual care of the chapel. The bones were placed in a wooden box covered in black velvet and decorated with the cross of Santiago, church records show.

Meanwhile, the cathedral itself underwent a thorough reconstruction and on July 4, 1606, the remains were moved into the new church, which was severely damaged by an earthquake in 1609. Sometime between 1623 and 1629 the bones were moved again, inside the church.

In 1661 a verification process took place for the remains of St. Toribio, destined to become Peru's first saint. In the records connected with St. Toribio, church documents mention a wooden box covered with brown velvet, enclosing a lead box with the inscription: "AQVÍ ESTÁ LA CABEÇA DEL SEÑOR MARQVÉS DON FRANCISCO PIZARO QVE DESCVBRIO Y GAÑO LOS REYNOS DEL PIRV Y PVSO EN LA REAL CORONA DE CASTILLA [Here is the skull of the Marquis Don Francisco Pizarro who discovered and won Peru and placed it under the crown of Castile]." More than two centuries later, this inscription would prove to be a crucial piece of evidence.

The cathedral was damaged anew in the earthquake of 1746. By 1778 a virtually new cathedral had been completed on the same site.

In 1891 came the three hundred and fiftieth anniversary of Pizarro's death, and for the first time a committee of scientists was appointed to examine the well-preserved, mummified body from the crypt under the altar of the cathedral that had been identified by church officials as that of Pizarro. This mummy, it should be made clear, was a natural mummy, preserved by the exceptional dryness of the air at Lima's high altitude; it was not, like an Egyptian mummy, artificially embalmed.

The source of the identification is an important detail: it was on the evidence of these priests and sacristans that the investigators relied. It was thought their testimony was unimpeachable, that they had carefully preserved Pizarro's body and his identification over the centuries, handing down the evidence in an unbroken chain. Surely they could not be mistaken! And so the investigators in 1891 began their examination with a strong prejudice in favor of the remains before them.

An American anthropologist, W. J. McGee, was present at the exhumation and wrote a full account of the proceedings for the *American Anthropologist,* Vol. VII, No. 1 (January 1894). The commission lavished great pains on the desiccated corpse, describing it inside out, inch by inch. Three pages of measurements are part of McGee's account.

The investigators were much struck by the fact that the mummy had no hands; that its skull was largely bare and exposed while dried flesh covered most of the rest of the body; that, even though it was male, it had no genitals; that there were gaping holes in the soft tissue at several points; and that, in their opinion, the skull looked like that of a criminal, with its jutting jaw and heavy-set base. It also seemed to possess an indented trench, known in those days as the "fossa of Lombroso," which takes its name from a celebrated Italian criminologist. Such fanciful terms are no longer accepted today.

"In prognathism, in the general conformation of the cranium, in the breadth and fullness of the basal and occipital regions of the brain-case, in the fossa of Lombroso, in all other important respects, the head is that of the typical criminal of to-day," McGee wrote decisively. Interestingly enough, this was viewed as yet another proof that the skull was indeed Pizarro's. Only a brute could have subdued Peru as bloodily as he did. Or, as McGee put it delicately, "The hero of history in earlier centuries is of rugged mold, and the heroism of the olden time is the crime of our softened lexicon. So Pizarro may well be judged as the representative of a class necessary and good in its age but not adjusted to the higher humanities of the present day."

The missing hands, the lopped-off genitals and the cavities in the soft tissue were blamed on the assassins. They must have mutilated Pizarro's dead body after they killed him. Corruption took hold in places where the skin had been pierced. Pizarro had been stabbed in the throat. From this wound, decay and maggots must have invaded the skull and stripped away its skin. The investigators concluded that, beyond the shadow of any doubt, these remains belonged to Pizarro. The mummy was blessed and then reverently reburied, with seals of authenticity attached to it by cotton cords and copper wires. The dusty innards were carefully collected and placed in a glass bottle, which was corked and deposited in the coffin. The remains of clothing surrounding the body were also carefully collected and wrapped up. Documents were prepared in triplicate, attesting that these were the true remains of the conquistador. A beautiful, ornate sarcophagus of glass, marble and bronze was constructed to hold the authenticated mummy. Over the years hundreds of thousands of people would pass by it, peer into it, and pay homage to it. On my first visit to Lima I saw people kneeling before it in silent prayer.

This state of affairs might have gone on indefinitely had not four workmen, who were cleaning the crypt beneath the altar one Friday in 1977, removed some bricks from a large, square, free-standing pilaster at the center of the crypt. In the exposed recess, they saw a flat, horizontal row of wooden planks. The workers said nothing to church officials of their find. Returning the next day, they removed more bricks and disclosed a second row of planks. Between these two planked floorings were two wooden boxes filled with human bones. Besides bones, one of the boxes held a lead casket on whose lid was an inscription, incised around the four edges: "AQVÍ ESTÁ LA CABEÇA DEL SEÑOR MARQVÉS DON FRANCISCO PIZARO . . ." it began, and the rest of the inscription was, word for word, identical with that seen and copied down by church officials in 1661.

This was an astonishing find. In the center of the lid of the lead box was a hexafoil pattern, a six-leafed design that some have taken as a veiled reference to the Star of David. Rumors had pursued Pizarro, in life and after death, that he came from a family of *conversos*, or forcibly converted Jews. This enigmatic six-leafed flower was a fascinating footnote to the discovery.

The workmen had hitherto kept silent about their discovery. One cannot help but suspect that if the casket had been made of silver it would have been stolen and melted down, and its contents lost forever. But when, after rubbing the metal, they found it was nothing more precious than lead, the men decided to inform church officials and get credit for the discovery. The authorities immediately called on Dr. Hugo Ludeña, a distinguished Peruvian historian, to investigate the matter. Ludeña in turn brought in other scholars: Dr. Pedro Weiss, an internationally known Peruvian physician and anthropologist who has a fascinating collection of Inca skulls; and two radiologists, Dr. Oscar Soto and his wife, Dr. Ladis Soto.

Ludeña, Weiss and the Sotos concurred in their opinion that the skull in the lead casket belonged to Pizarro, but their findings were hotly disputed by other Peruvian scholars, who insisted the mummy in the glass sarcophagus had to be genuine. Dr. Ludeña approached Dr. Robert Benfer, a colleague of mine who teaches anthropology at the University of Missouri and who has excavated many prehistoric Peruvian burials, asking him to look at the remains. Bob suggested that I collaborate because of my forensic experience. I made two trips to Lima in early 1984 to examine the bones and, on July 4, 1984, we also participated in the opening of the sarcophagus, the removal of the mummy and its examination in the cathedral library.

Of the two wooden boxes found in the hidden niche, the larger one, which we called Box A, contained the mixed remains of several skeletons: among them were the remains of at least two children, an elderly female, the skull and postcranial remains of an elderly male and the skull-less, postcranial skeleton of a second elderly male. There were also the rusty remnants of a sword. This box was lined with tatters of brown velvet and had an outline of a cross upon it. The cross itself was long gone, but the nails to attach it remained, and these were found to contain the rather rare metal, vanadium. They were probably made of melted-down sword steel.

The second wooden box, referred to as Box B, was painted light green and its interior was coated with a kind of red plaster. This, too, contained human bones, as well as the lead container with the inscription, inside which was found a human skull. This skull fitted nicely to the skull-less remains of the elderly male found in the other box. Its occipital condyles, the part of the skull's base where it joins the neck, were perfectly congruent with the uppermost vertebrae of the skeleton in Box A. It appeared that the owner of this skull had lost a good many teeth before he died, including most of his upper molars and many of the incisors and molars of the lower jaw. This reunited skull and skeleton belonged to a white male at least sixty years old at the time of his death, who stood about sixty-five to sixty-nine inches tall in life, based on the length of his long bones.

(Because Pizarro was a foundling, his age at the time of his death is doubtful. He was variously said to be sixty-three or sixty-five years old by contemporary historians.)

When Bob and I examined the skull and other bones carefully, we began to see clear traces of terrible wounds. There were no fewer than four sword thrusts to the neck. In one, a double-edged weapon had entered the neck from the right side and nicked the first cervical vertebra. The direction of the sword thrust was clear: it would have pierced the right vertebral artery. This was a mortal blow. A second sword thrust, also from the right, was equally devastating: it had cut away portions of vertebrae and the blade had been pressed home with tremendous force. A third thrust to the neck nearly split open the spinal cord. A fourth passed through the right vertebral opening of another neckbone and would also have cut through the right vertebral artery.

As Bob and I followed the backbone down into the trunk, we saw other injuries. The sixth thoracic vertebra clearly showed the marks of a stab wound from a blade thrust downward into the body at an angle of fifteen degrees. A second thrust pierced the abdomen and nicked the twelfth thoracic vertebra. The ninth right rib was also nicked, but the rib cortex was crumbly and we were not able to determine whether this nick was due to a stab wound. The development of the spine in general, with characteristic pockmarks and herniations, showed that it belonged to a man who had lived a long, vigorous life.

There were also wounds in the arms and hands of the skeleton, the sort of injuries we call "defensive wounds," which are suffered when someone tries to defend himself with his hands. The right humerus, or upper arm, had been cut cleanly and obliquely by an edged weapon. Probably a heavy sword, not a rapier, had been used here, in an attempt to disable the man whose skeleton lay before us. There were two deep nicks on the left first metacarpal bone of the hand, below the thumb. The right fifth metacarpal bone had been broken off altogether and was not in the box. It may have been broken off when Pizarro was disarmed.

The right lower armbone, or ulna, showed an old fracture that indicated the owner had broken his arm as a boy. Greenish stains were found on some of the heelbones, which agreed with the story that Pizarro had been buried with a single Moorish spur. The green was probably verdigris, from copper in the spur. From the relative size of the bumps on the bones where muscles had been attached, it was clear that the individual had been right-handed. Many of the joints showed "lipping," which is associated with arthritis. We know Pizarro found it painful to ride a horse, preferring to walk instead. The size of the bones showed they belonged in life to a well-developed, robust man.

The lower jaw, or mandible, had fallen away from the skull as it usually does after death. On its lower margin, beneath the chin, were eleven finely incised marks, clearly made by sharp, double-edged weapons pointing in several directions. One of these marks lined up perfectly with one of the deeper stab wounds found in the neck, thus furnishing more proof that the skull in the leaden coffer truly belonged with the set of loose bones in the other box. These telltale nicks indicated that the deceased had either been stabbed repeatedly through the neck or, more probably, that one assailant had thrust his sword in, then sawed the blade back and forth against the jawbone, aiming upward into the neck and head and scratching the mandible in the process.

The skull, too, showed signs of trauma. There was a clean fracture or cut through the right zygomatic arch of the skull, a kind of slender bridge of bone that runs back from the cheekbone on both sides of our heads. This may have been caused by a sword thrust. Another thrust had passed through the left eye socket and left a clear nick in the bone where it exited from the left wall of the orbit. A rapier or dagger had passed into the brain through the neck, up into the right base of the skull, where it had been twisted and thrust in again. The sphenoid bone on the left side of the skull base showed signs of yet another pair of thrusts. Yet in spite of all these stabbings, the braincase was remarkably intact. The high nasal bridge showed clear evidence of an old fracture that had healed; the owner of the skeleton had broken his nose earlier in his violent life.

All in all, the skull and skeletal remains before me were unmistakably those of a man who had suffered a dreadful, violent death. His assailants had stabbed him over and over again, concentrating their homicidal fury on his head and neck. There were at least eleven stab wounds made by the points of weapons on the bones—possibly as many as fourteen. There were as many as fourteen separate cuts made by sharp edges on the bones and one possible blunt-force fracture of the hand. Interestingly, most of the wounds were on the right side of the body and neck. This is the side a right-handed swordsman would present to his opponents. The extraordinary trauma inflicted on the neck agreed very closely with accounts of Pizarro's murder. The angle of some of the wounds suggested that they were inflicted as the victim lay on the floor. The defensive wounds to the hands and arm show that the victim vainly struggled to push away the plunging swords. His last sight on earth must have been terrible: flashing steel points, rising and falling and piercing his body, his head, his throat and his left eye. Death, when it came at last, must have been a merciful release.

It should also be noted that not every stab wound will leave a mark on the skeleton underneath. In one of my modern cases, the skin of a murdered man revealed twenty-four separate stab wounds, yet only eight of these left marks on his skeleton. It is very likely that Pizarro was stabbed many more times than his bones disclose.

The other bones found in Box A could not be identified with certainty. The two children may have been Pizarro's sons, Juan and Gonzalo, who are said to have died at the ages of four and ten respectively. The dental remains of the older child's skeleton placed his age at between eight and eleven years. The remains of the younger child showed him to be about two years old, both dentally and skeletally. We can only guess about the female remains. Perhaps they are those of Doña Inés Muñoz, the wife of the faithful Alcántara, who died fighting for his chief. Perhaps the remains of the second elderly male are those of Alcántara himself. We cannot tell.

The wounds and the inscription on the lead box containing the skull made it clear beyond any doubt that we were dealing with the remains of Pizarro. One question remained: who was the mummy in the glass coffin upstairs?

Bob and I were shown into the sumptuous cathedral library, with its beautifully paneled walls, its gorgeous old leather-bound volumes and its wealth of silver and gold crucifixes and religious paintings. Amid this splendor, on a table, lay the leathery old mummy, its skin greasy to the touch, and with a single dried eyeball lying deep within one shadowy socket of its fleshless face. Its head had been separated from its body in 1891 and wired back on.

We photographed and measured the mummy carefully. Despite the absence of genitals, we were able to determine easily that it was a male of advanced years, who had been 165.5 cm (about five feet, five inches) tall in life. The skeletal morphology was rather effeminate or "gracile," as we call it: the man had been something of a physical weakling in life. The skin of the legs bore the marks of high stockings which had long since disappeared, and the marks of some cord used long ago to bind the legs together. The pattern of the velvet sarcophagus liner was etched into the skin of the back.

Every remaining bit of skin on the mummy was minutely examined for evidence of wounds. There were none. The exposed bones were examined carefully with various magnifying devices. We found absolutely no evidence of unhealed fractures, chips, scratches or incised marks. The bone was in excellent condition and any damage caused by trauma would have been clearly evident. None could be seen.

The conclusion was inescapable: we were dealing with an impostor. The man who lay before us was no soldier. He had lived a quiet life and had died a quiet death. Most likely he was a churchman, a scholar or a petty functionary of the government whose remains had somehow got confounded with Pizarro's in the earthquake-ridden centuries after the conquistador's death. It is certainly amusing that the 1891 investigators thought his skull was that of a criminal! So much for the "fossa of Lombroso" and all such quackeries!

A careful cast was made of Pizarro's skull by Robert Levy of the Florida Museum of Natural History, and from it Betty Pat Gatliff of SKULLpture Inc., an Oklahoma firm specializing in such reconstructions, was able to build up a clay bust of Francisco Pizarro as he looked in life: a heavy-set man with a broad, peasant's face. This bust was presented to the museum of the Convent of La Coria in Pizarro's native city, Trujillo, Spain, along with a cast of the skull from the lead casket in Lima.

Pizarro's bones were placed where they belonged, inside the glass-walled sarcophagus in the cathedral chapel, where they can still be seen today. The impostor mummy, when last I saw him, was lying ignobly on a piece of plywood propped between two sawhorses in the cathedral crypt, destined for an anonymous reburial in the bow-

els of the cathedral. Whoever he was, he cannot complain. For
nearly a hundred years he had basked in the borrowed glory of
Francisco Pizarro. He was knelt before, prayed to and well-nigh
worshiped by thousands of pilgrims. He enjoyed far more homage
than most of us receive after death, and with this flood of fervent,
mistaken devotion his ghost must rest content. Fame is fleeting—
even in death.

Arsenic and "Old Rough and Ready"

Duncan is in his grave;
After life's fitful fever he sleeps well;
Treason has done his worst: nor steel, nor poison,
Malice domestic, foreign levy, nothing,
Can touch him further. . . .

—Shakespeare, *Macbeth*, Act III, Scene 2

Summers in Washington, D.C., can be horribly hot, and July 4, 1850, was infernal. President Zachary Taylor, hero of the Battle of Buena Vista in the Mexican War, had just returned from a ceremony in the blazing sun, at which he laid the foundation-stone for the Washington Monument. He was tired, hungry and thirsty. He wolfed down a big meal of raw vegetables, fresh cherries and iced buttermilk. Within a very short time it became apparent that the food had not agreed with him. The President developed gastroenteritis and acute diarrhea and was forced to take to his bed. Five days later, on July 9, the man known to his contemporaries as "Old Rough and Ready" was dead. He was sixty-six years old and had been President just sixteen months.

Taylor's abrupt death came at a crucial point in American history. It removed from the scene a man whose force of character might have quelled the storm brewing across America over slavery— or hastened that storm's breaking. Taylor might have recalled his fellow Southerners to a sense of the duty they owed to their country; but it is equally possible that he might have driven them to desperate deeds by opposing them with naked force. We can never know. A single ill-digested meal toppled Taylor into his grave; the rest is guesswork and silence.

Some historians have called Zachary Taylor the Dwight Eisenhower of his day, because of his brilliant military record; but there was an element of fire, of hot-tempered truculence, in Taylor that was wholly missing from Ike's serene, controlled disposition. A Southerner who owned sugar and cotton plantations worked by over four hundred slaves—his daughter, Knox, was the first wife of the man who would become president of the Confederacy, Jefferson Davis, and his son, Richard, served as a general for the South in the Civil War—Taylor nevertheless campaigned hard to admit California and New Mexico as free states and threatened to lead an army in person against any Southerners who would not submit to laws enacted by Congress. When two Southern legislators, Alexander Stephens and Robert Toombs, told Taylor he was betraying the South, the President exploded, saying he would hang all "traitors" to the Union with no more compunction than he had shown when hanging spies and deserters in Mexico. In the days immediately preceding his fatal illness, Taylor ordered the military garrison of Santa Fe, New Mexico, to be reinforced against possible attacks by proslavery militiamen from Texas. He was a tough man, singularly unafraid of his enemies, willing to do battle to keep the United States one nation, indivisible.

His death marked an important crossroads in the crisis over slavery. His successor, Millard Fillmore, was at pains to mollify the angry Southerners whom Taylor had defied. The new President quietly shelved New Mexico's application for statehood and lent his support to a jellified compromise bill that contained all sorts of sops

224

to satisfy both sides of the slavery question. The outbreak of the Civil War was postponed for another decade, and in the awful glare of that cataclysmic passage of arms, the story of Zachary Taylor, his short presidency and his sudden death, receded into oblivion. Few schoolchildren today could name the twelfth President of the United States. The bumbling Millard Fillmore is better known than the hard-bitten hero of Buena Vista.

Yet from time to time Taylor's sudden death would tax the ingenuity of amateur historians. Aged sixty-six, he was old but not decrepit. His constitution had been tried and tempered in arduous campaigns in Mexico, and earlier in Florida against the Seminole Indians. He was no stranger to heat and thirst. Could raw vegetables and fruit, washed down with cold milk, kill a man? Books published in 1928 and again in 1940 raised the possibility that Taylor had been poisoned by proslavery conspirators. If so, he, not Abraham Lincoln, would have been the first President in American history to be assassinated.

My mind was far from these theories in 1991, when I received a visit from Clare Rising in the office I then occupied in the Florida Museum of Natural History. Rising was one of our alumnae: she had received her Ph.D. in English from the University of Florida and was the prize-winning author of *Season of the Wild Rose,* a historical novel set during the Civil War. It was while researching this novel that she had come across the Taylor case, and it had fascinated her ever since. She was writing a book about Taylor. She described his symptoms—vomiting, abdominal spasms, diarrhea and progressive weakening—which she had gleaned from contemporary accounts of his death. Was it possible, she asked me, that such symptoms might result from poisoning?

I told Rising that I wasn't a pathologist but that the symptoms she had described certainly could have resulted from arsenic poisoning.

She said: "Well, could this be proven?" And I explained that arsenic and other metallic poisons are quickly deposited in the skeletal system and hair of poisoning victims, if they live for a few days after the initial intake of the poison. Such metals would remain in the hair and bones, even after death.

She asked: "How could this be proven?" I told her it would be a fairly simple matter, given access to the remains, to have tests done that would prove the presence or absence of arsenic.

I gradually discovered that Rising was an extremely persistent and single-minded individual. Initially I had scant interest in the Taylor question, and I tried to steer her toward other people in the field who I felt were perfectly competent to conduct such tests. I suggested she contact my colleague, Doug Ubelaker, at the Smithsonian Institution. I suggested the Armed Forces Institute of Pathology at Walter Reed Hospital. I suggested the Armed Forces Medical Museum. I furnished her with names and telephone numbers.

In vain. Rising kept returning to me. She had a scholarly obsession with Zachary Taylor—"my Zachary," she called him fondly—and she saw this inquiry as a way to do justice to a rather neglected figure in American history. I was less sanguine than she. Moreover the enormity of exhuming a former President of the United States was somewhat daunting. I had assisted at many exhumations, but never at one of such extraordinary historical significance. I had no misgivings about the technical side of the affair. No corpse on earth has the power to overawe me. Our defunct bodies are all equal before science. Nevertheless, I could dimly foresee how controversial this project might prove, and what a fanfaronade of media attention might accompany it. As events were to show, my fears proved justified many times over!

Finally, on the latest of her many visits, Rising sat down in a chair across from my desk and said: "Well, just how would we get permission?"

I explained to her something that many people do not know: human remains are not the property of cemeteries. They don't belong to the nation, no matter who they were in life. Nor do they belong to the courts. They belong to the relatives who survive them.

From a legal standpoint, dead human bodies are treated exactly the same as any other personal effects left behind by the deceased. They are passed on, together with the rest of the estate. You own the remains of your dead ancestors. They are yours by law.

Therefore, I told Rising, if anyone wanted to examine a body, the first step must be to approach the surviving family members. These in turn can request a funeral director licensed in the state to open the grave, provided the body is properly reburied upon completion of the examination. I told her that very often in murder cases we go through this procedure, with the families' permission. If the family agrees, we need not go through the courts. This timesaving procedure is especially useful when we are dealing with murder victims who are buried in states other than those where the murders took place.

Rising was elated. She told me she had tracked down many of the living relatives and knew from genealogies who the nearest direct descendant was—and she mentioned a man in Louisiana whose name is familiar to millions of people.

I said: "Well, all you have to do is get that gentleman to sign a request that the nearest licensed funeral director open the tomb."

I have already said Rising was persistent. But even I was surprised when she triumphantly telephoned me from Louisiana a few weeks later and announced that she had won permission to exhume the remains of Zachary Taylor. Not only that: she had already approached a funeral director in Louisville, Kentucky, whose firm had moved President Taylor and his wife from an older mausoleum to a newer aboveground tomb in the 1920s. Rising's enthusiasm was contagious. The funeral director said that he would not only cooperate but would perform the exhumation without charge.

Zachary Taylor, I learned, was entombed in the Zachary Taylor National Cemetery in Louisville, Kentucky, which, like all national cemeteries, is supervised by the Veterans Administration. The land for that cemetery had been donated to the federal government by the Taylor family, but they had retained ownership of a strip of land at the rear of the cemetery, on both sides of the Taylor mausoleum, as a private family burial plot. Everything else was under VA stewardship.

I did some soul-searching before agreeing to be present at the exhumation. It is my firm belief that the dead have a right to privacy and that there must be a good, compelling reason for us to break in upon the slumber of the grave. In the case of President Taylor, there was the charge—albeit unproven—of murder, the foulest crime man can commit. For over a hundred and forty years it had hovered around Taylor's memory like a miasma. Now we were in a position to decide once and for all whether or not there was anything to it. The relatives had given their consent. Their scruples had been satisfied that this was a legitimate inquiry, and not an exercise in idle speculation. The local coroner, Dr. Richard Greathouse, had agreed to treat the procedure as an official investigation into the cause of Taylor's death, and he had enlisted the aid of the state medical examiner, Dr. George Nichols IV.

It was the consent of the relatives, however, that weighed most with me. If they saw no indignity in exhuming Taylor, then there was none. Rising had written to family members as far away as Rome and Stockholm, and all had consented to the investigation. The *New York Times* editorialized that our inquiry showed "a cavalier contempt for the dead," but I could not agree. It would be frivolous indeed to exhume a President to see if he had suffered from a certain disease, or to learn some small particular about his life and times. But murder is another thing entirely, and murder was what we aimed to prove or disprove.

The team I had put together consisted of myself, Dr. Nichols, Dr. William Hamilton, the District 8 medical examiner in Florida, who had worked for Dr. Nichols before coming to Gainesville (and who had experience in examining the exhumed victims of arsenic poisoning), two graduate students, Arlene Albert and Dana Austin-Smith, who would do the still photography, and a local retired attorney and historian, Bill Goza, who would lend us historical assistance and expedite details. Finally, my wife Margaret, a media specialist who is always an important member of my team, would handle logistics and take care of videotaping the investigation for scientific purposes.

A date was set. We made hotel reservations and rented a van for the following weekend. Then difficulties began to crop up. Rising telephoned me, saying that a problem had arisen with the Veterans Administration. The VA was reluctant to give permission for the exhumation. When I finally reached a high-level official in the VA, he said the matter might have to be resolved at "a higher level."

I said: "What do you mean by 'higher'?"

And he said: "Since it involves the remains of a President, the White House."

By now it was Thursday. The tomb was supposed to be opened the next Monday. There was no way we could secure presidential permission in that short interval. Even though the Taylor family owned the mausoleum and the strip of land adjacent to it, the VA ran the cemetery and had the key to the Taylor crypt. The Zachary Taylor mausoleum was situated at the back of the cemetery, and the VA controlled all the land in front of it. They could simply lock the front gate and there would be little we could do to oppose them.

With some disappointment—for by now I had become rather interested in this project—I phoned Rising and said there was no way we could proceed the following Monday. Perhaps some other time . . . In the meantime all our arrangements were canceled.

Shortly afterward, Rising called me back and said she'd been in contact with the coroner, Dr. Richard Greathouse. He, I discovered, wasn't about to be dictated to by the Veterans Administration. He was a man of extraordinary determination, confidence and a strong sense of territory. Greathouse told Rising to tell me that whether I came to Louisville or stayed home was all the same to him. I was welcome to be on hand if I liked. But with or without me, Zachary Taylor's tomb was going to be opened that Monday morning and the only way the federal government could prevent this was by armed force!

So, after reassembling all our broken travel arrangements, we left for Louisville on Saturday morning. We arrived Sunday afternoon at the hotel, a Ramada Inn located right beside the Zachary Taylor National Cemetery. As we pulled into the parking lot we were horrified to see a host of satellite dishes, mounted on large vehicles, surrounding the hotel. When I checked into the hotel I learned to my chagrin that I had telephone messages waiting for me from the "Today" show, "Good Morning America," CNN and various other news organizations. Rising met us at the hotel and told us the VA desired a meeting with us right away.

The VA was worried about publicity and I didn't blame them: the whole Taylor exhumation was fast becoming a media circus. The VA was no longer opposed to exhuming Taylor, but it was adamantly opposed to taking pictures of the remains. "No photos," the two representatives told us firmly.

I explained that as forensic scientists we were obligated to document what we did and that we couldn't proceed without photographs.

The VA official said: "How do we know these photographs won't show up in the *National Enquirer?*"

"Easy," I answered him. "Show me one photograph I've ever taken that has appeared in any newspaper or magazine or publication such as the *National Enquirer.*" I explained that the photos would be used in scientific books, publications and scientific articles. This appeared to satisfy him.

That Sunday evening was one of the most interesting and atmospheric of my life. We went to a reception and dinner at Zachary Taylor's old home, which is located not far behind the cemetery. It is a splendid old dwelling and its owners are devoted to the President's memory. They have delved into every aspect of his life with extraordinary zeal. Other members of the Taylor family were there, including the President's two great-great-great-great-granddaughters, a beautiful and vivacious pair of young women who charmed everyone with their lively, sparkling manner. I was amazed to hear that, had the VA forbidden us access, the Taylor family had made arrangements with neighbors whose property abutted the rear of the cemetery, to climb over the wall and enter the mausoleum directly from behind! I was silently relieved matters had not gone so far.

Dinner was served in a gorgeous dining room overhung by magnificent chandeliers. Portraits of Zachary Taylor hung everywhere, and the elegant meal was concluded by a dessert of pecan pie that was said to be an old family recipe, a favorite of the President's. Margaret's health was toasted—it was her birthday—and we both learned wonderful bits of Taylor family lore and heard many fascinating anecdotes about "Old Rough and Ready" from the lips of those to whom he was no remote textbook figure, but a beloved and well-remembered ancestor. Seldom has history come so agreeably to life as it did for me that evening.

Yet at the back of everyone's mind was the dark and fascinating prospect of the next day. We were about to resurrect a dead man, yet the mood was lively, convivial, even festive. There was an indefinable air of keen anticipation: tomorrow morning the President whose likeness hung upon the walls of this dining room, Zachary Taylor himself, would reenter the world of the living. He would step back onto the stage of American history he had suddenly vacated a hundred and forty-one years earlier.

The next morning, whatever hopes we had that the investigation in the cemetery would be conducted quietly and decorously were dashed. When we arrived at the entrance to the cemetery at 9 A.M. we found the fire department at the front gate, directing traffic. Police were everywhere. The main avenue of the cemetery was lined with hundreds of people. Media camera units were positioned in cherry-picker cranes overhead. We were let through a police barrier and parked on the curved drive just in front of the Taylor tomb. Watched by thousands of inquisitive eyes, we unloaded our equipment and proceeded to document the area.

The local funeral director had secured services of some volunteers from a memorial vault company to assist in the delicate task of moving the massive slab of Tennessee marble that sealed the vault containing the coffins of President and Mrs. Taylor. This enormous vault was inside the tomb, with only a couple of feet of clearance on three sides.

When the slab was lifted, a badly rotted wooden casket was seen to be lying within the vault. Inside this casket was a lead liner, all the seams of which had been soldered shut. Under closer examination, we saw a rectangular soldered plate near the head of the liner. Beneath this plate was a cracked glass window. The apparent purpose of this glass window was to allow the dead President to be viewed while lying in state in his coffin at the White House.

We had not expected to find this sealed box of lead and had no tools with which to open it. In any case the mausoleum was so small that there was no room to work or maneuver, and the milling crowds outside were oppressive. We decided to take the lead liner and the enclosed remains to the office of the state medical examiner and to open it there.

Now we were alone at last, and now the true investigation could begin. At the office of the medical examiner, we changed to scrub suits and discussed how the lead liner could best be opened. It looked solid, but we now saw it was pocked with several perforations. Historical records said Taylor had not been embalmed—his wife had forbidden it. Instead, his body had been packed in ice for the lying in state. As his body decomposed within the lead box, the resultant butyric acids had eaten through the metal in several places. So these holes were an important piece of evidence. Because they showed Taylor had not been embalmed, and because arsenic was part of the nineteenth-century embalming process, we could be sure the remains had not been contaminated by an undertaker.

But how to open the box? Initially it was decided to use a small blowtorch. A worker from the maintenance department of the county coroner's office was summoned to the room and, using a small torch attached to a miniature propane tank, he began carefully to melt the solder joints of the casket. Suddenly I had a horrifying thought. Peering through the opened portion of the seam, I could see that the box was lined with cloth! If this cloth liner should catch fire from the flame of the blowtorch, our proposed examination of Zachary Taylor might end with his unexpected cremation! The blowtorch was extinguished instantly and sent back to the basement.

We considered awhile and then fell back on a trusty Stryker saw, the oscillating bladed tool that is used to cut bone in autopsies. This saw went through the lead liner like cheese, and the top popped off as neatly as if we had used a can opener.

The lid was moved out of the way and all of us peered down into the depths of the container. There lay all that remained of President Zachary Taylor.

The former President had been totally skeletonized. Abundant hair could be seen adhering to the skull. The deceased President's bushy eyebrows were still visible, clinging to the supraorbital ridges above his skull's eye sockets. The hair was dark, flecked with gray. For the rest, he presented an austere picture of simple mortality: a skeleton, clad in his funeral attire, his skull pillowed on a bunch of straw stuffed beneath the casket liner. He had one missing tooth and one collapsed crown, but otherwise his teeth were still magnificent. Taylor must have had a brilliant, winning smile in life.

The deceased President was dressed in an unusual one-piece suit that consisted of a pleated shirtlike top with buttoned sleeves, and plain trousers below. I suppose it was the nineteenth-century equivalent of a jumpsuit, all of one piece and probably chosen for convenience's sake. He wore no shoes or stockings, but his bony hands were sheathed in fine cloth gloves. Under his fallen lower jaw there was a very large cloth bow tie knotted butterfly fashion around his neck, a beautiful and curiously soft-looking thing, almost the sort of adornment a girl might wear.

All of the clothing and gloves must have been white originally, but now they were yellowed with age and stained by the decomposition process to a tobacco-like brown. As I have already mentioned, the lead liner itself had a cloth lining which was a faint beige color, falling down in several places. The darkness of the hair may have been due to decomposition. Apart from a few lumps of adipocere, a waxy substance that forms when body fats combine with moisture, the remains were entirely skeletal.

Then we went to work. Photographs were taken. A forensic dentist examined the teeth. With a pair of scissors I carefully cut the back of the gloves down each finger and removed all ten fingernails. I gently collected sufficient samples of hair from the President's head and his body. In the area of the feet I found several fallen toenails, including both of the nails from the great toes. We also sampled a small portion of bone from the breastbone or sternum, took a small piece of the adipocere and collected samples of the textiles from under the body that had soaked up fluids from the decomposing remains. If arsenic had been used to kill Taylor, arsenic would be present in all these things.

All the samples were placed in envelopes. Everything was divided—fingernails, hair, adipocere, bone, fabrics—so that we had two identical sets of samples. One set of specimens went to the Oak Ridge National Laboratory for analysis and the other to the Kentucky laboratory that routinely performs toxicology work for the state medical examiner.

By now it was around 4 P.M. The examination was nearly complete. The coroner's office was telephoning around Louisville to find a specialist in soldering lead. At length a man who worked with lead roofs was located and agreed to come to the office and solder the lead box shut again.

Before he arrived, Taylor's two great-great-great-great-granddaughters asked to see their ancestor. This was a delicate situation. I have already described the skeletal state of the remains. Gently we described the contents of the lead box to them, and asked again: were they quite sure they wanted to look? They insisted they did, they assured us they could stand the sight. So at length the two young women were allowed to come into the room and peer into the casket containing their renowned forebear. They were enthralled, not in the least upset. I still have a photograph of them in the room, gesturing with animation and smiling excitedly.

Clare Rising, who had devoted so much time to explicating the Taylor riddle, was also permitted to come in and have a brief glimpse of the deceased President. She approached the casket with considerable hesitation and no little awe. I fixed my eyes on her and I could sense that, at that moment, she wasn't looking at a mere mass of dead bones. She was gazing on the legendary figure of history: Zachary Taylor.

The container was closed, returned to the cemetery with an American flag draped around it. It was replaced in the vault and the heavy marble lid was replaced. This time the marble was sealed with epoxy that would guarantee the Taylors' privacy and repose. After this, we all went home to await the results of the laboratory analysis.

Shortly after I returned to Gainesville, the results were released by Dr. Nichols's office. They were clear and unequivocal. The amounts of arsenic found in all samples were consistent throughout. They showed that President Taylor had in his remains only the levels of arsenic consistent with any person who lived in the nineteenth century. The levels were in every case minuscule. They could never have produced death, or even illness.

Arsenic is a remarkable and powerful poison that can kill quickly or slowly, depending on the dosage. A sudden, massive dose of arsenic could kill within hours and, if this occurs, no trace of the poison will be deposited in the hair or nails or bones of the deceased. But if the victim lives for twenty-eight to thirty hours after ingesting the arsenic, minute traces of the poison will be deposited in the hair and bones. As we all know, Zachary Taylor lived for five days after the onset of his symptoms. There was ample time for arsenic to be deposited in his system, if he had been poisoned. Our investigation demonstrated, once and for all, that he hadn't.

It is remotely possible that another poison might have been used to kill Taylor, but only arsenic would have produced the symptoms he showed before dying, and arsenic was by now conclusively out of the question. The verdict of history must be that Zachary Taylor died of natural causes. Indeed, he may have been unwittingly killed by his doctors.

In those days, cathartics and laxatives were prescribed for diarrhea, and fluids were often deliberately withheld, on the advice of doctors. A strong case might be made that the President had a fairly routine case of intestinal infection. Perhaps the vegetables and cherries he devoured had not been washed, or had been washed in contaminated water. The heat of July would have afforded a fertile breeding ground for *E. coli* germs and these, massed in millions in his gut, may have formed an army the old general could not defeat.

One minor note: we also found in the coffin several pupa cases of flies that were attracted to the dead President in that hot summer so long ago. These bold insects had paid a price for their temerity: their offspring had been buried alive with the illustrious man their parents had presumed to light upon.

The aftermath was all very anticlimactic. I learned, if I did not already know, how fickle was the fancy of the American media. Zachary Taylor the Murder Victim was news. Zachary Taylor the President who died a natural death was history, and ancient history at that. The satellite dishes were stowed, the camera lenses were capped, the generators were unplugged, the notebooks snapped shut. No more did the networks jangle my phone, wooing me with their blandishments. "Old Rough and Ready" resumed his interrupted sleep, and I returned to my modern murders unmolested. Like hoarfrost at noon, the media simply evanesced.

Clare Rising finished her book on Zachary Taylor, but as far as I know it remains unpublished, despite her past literary success. She clung to her poisoning theory and did extensive additional research in the medical literature, trying to explain why, even though Taylor might have been poisoned, no poison would show up in a chemical analysis. But to my mind the death of President Taylor has been settled now, and Clare Rising is entitled to some of the credit whether she agrees or not. Without her extraordinary efforts, the mystery might have lingered indefinitely. Now it is resolved.

Zachary Taylor can take his proper place in history, as a military commander who fought hard for his country and as a President who did not shrink from his duty. His last hours may have been uncomfortable, but they were not unnatural. He was not assassinated. And, like the big soft bow tie he wore in his coffin, the old President did have a gentler side.

It was Zachary Taylor who coined the term "First Lady." He used these words to describe Dolly Madison at her funeral in 1849: "She will never be forgotten, because she was truly our first lady for a half century." This sincere piece of gallantry is among his smaller monuments. It came from Zachary Taylor's own heart—a heart that was gone, together with the storm and strife it struggled to master, long before the old President and I met.

The Tsar of All the Russias

"The world will never know what we did with them. . . ."

—Peter Voikov, Soviet ambassador to Poland, 1935

It was a sunny day on the edge of Siberia when I climbed the stairs to the second floor of the Forensic-Medical Examination Bureau, where the skeletons were kept. The bureau was located in Ekaterinburg, eight hundred miles from Moscow, deep in the Ural Mountains. A city of dreadful fame, Ekaterinburg is the Golgotha of Soviet Communism. Here, in the basement of a house that has since been destroyed, was carried out one of the most fateful mass executions in this century.

In Ekaterinburg, on the night of July 16–17, 1918, Tsar Nicholas II, the last of the Romanovs, was summoned downstairs with his whole family to a basement room in the so-called "House of Special Designation," a mansion requisitioned from an engineer named Ipatiev. Waiting for him was a Bolshevik death squad led by Commander Jacob Yurovsky.

Near midnight a decree of execution was read out to the amazed royal family and their servants: Tsar Nicholas, the Tsarina Alexandra, their frail hemophiliac son Alexei, their four daughters, Olga, Tatiana, Marie and Anastasia, the family doctor, Sergei Botkin, a cook named Kharitonov, a footman named Trupp and a maid named Anna Demidova—eleven people in all.

Yurovsky had not finished speaking when the first shots exploded in the narrow room. Thrown backward by the force of bullets, the Tsar spun around and fell dead. His family and retainers fell with him, in a blizzard of lead. The roar of a Fiat truck engine, running loudly outside the back door, helped mask the homicidal racket. Twenty minutes later the corpses were carried out into the summer night, where they vanished, seemingly forever.

"The world will never know what we did with them," boasted Peter Voikov, a Bolshevik official at Ekaterinburg who was ambassador to Poland when he uttered these words, seventeen years later.

On July 19 the local *Ural Worker* newspaper announced that the Tsar was dead:

EXECUTION OF NICHOLAS, THE BLOODY CROWNED MURDERER
SHOT WITHOUT BOURGEOIS FORMALITIES
BUT IN ACCORDANCE WITH OUR NEW DEMOCRATIC PRINCIPLES.

But no mention was made of his family, and for nearly three quarters of a century the exact details of the massacre remained a Soviet secret. Despite the most zealous searches by pro-Tsarist investigators immediately after the shootings, the corpses of the Tsar and his family were not unearthed. Only a single finger, apparently belonging to a woman, together with scattered burned and molten personal effects, turned up in the recesses of an abandoned mine twelve miles outside of the city.

Now, unexpectedly, from a bog on the outskirts of Ekaterinburg nine more or less complete skeletons had come to light in a shallow grave, along with fourteen bullets, bits of rope and a shattered jar that once contained sulfuric acid. Could these be the remains of the Romanovs? I and my colleagues had been invited by the Russians to come halfway around the world to try to answer this question.

Up a flight of stairs, down a long corridor—there was the entrance to the makeshift morgue. I recall the layout clearly. At the end of a long hallway on the second floor there is a wrought-iron gate. Behind this lies a metal door with some very impressive locks and wax seals. The room is behind this door.

Then our Russian hosts opened the door and said to us cheerfully: "Go to it."

We were let into a square room with two windows and a cluster of three desks at the center. Along all four walls at the edge of the room were long tables, about thirty inches wide, covered with white sheets.

On the sheets, lying head to toe around the room, were nine skeletons.

For me, these remains possessed a special fascination. I had first read of the Romanov murders forty-four years previously, as an eleven-year-old boy, in *Seven League Boots,* a 1935 book by the globetrotting journalist Richard Halliburton. Halliburton recounted how he had gone to Sverdlovsk, as Ekaterinburg was renamed by the Bolsheviks, and tracked down one of the Tsar's assassins, Peter Zacharovitch Ermakov, a brutal man known as "Comrade Mauser."

Coughing, spitting up blood, apparently dying of throat cancer, Ermakov told Halliburton a blood-freezing tale of wholesale murder:

"It was on July 12 that we had our final meeting and got our orders. We set the night of July 16th for the shooting—four days later," Ermakov said. "I had to make all the plans myself for the destruction of the bodies. We wanted to do the thing as quietly as possible, to be sure the Romanoffs didn't suspect in advance. And I wanted to make doubly sure that the bodies would be thoroughly destroyed. I didn't want the Whites to find a single bone." In July 1918 the White Russians were besieging Ekaterinburg and its fall was expected at any moment.

Ermakov said he spent the fourteenth reconnoitering the territory around Ekaterinburg for a suitable disposal site for the bodies. He settled on an abandoned mineshaft about twelve miles outside of town. His commander, Jacob Yurovsky, approved the site, Ermakov said.

"Next morning, we took an army truck and carried several big tins of gasoline out to one of the deepest mines. I also sent along two big buckets of sulphuric acid and a truckload of firewood. One of my soldiers stood guard over these supplies to frighten off any curious peasants who might be wandering around."

A driver was ordered to park his truck in front of the back door of the Ipatiev house and leave the engine running at full throttle. The noise of the engine, it was hoped, would drown the crack of gunshots.

"Vaganof was always with me. He was a good Bolshevik who hated the Tsar as much as I did. We could count on him to shoot straight!

"Yurovsky had a Nagant repeater. Vaganof and I had Mausers. We each carried twenty extra rounds of ammunition. . . . There were to be just we three executioners.

"That afternoon, we looked all over the house for a good place to do the shooting, and decided on the basement guard room. Being below ground, the shots wouldn't sound so loud. It was the right size too—about 18 feet long and 12 wide.

"If there were more than three of us, we'd be in each other's way."

At about midnight Yurovsky knocked on the Tsar's door and told him he and his family were to be evacuated because fighting had broken out on the outskirts of Ekaterinburg. The Tsar and his family took about an hour to prepare themselves.

"The door opened and the Tsar came out carrying Alexei. They both had on military caps and jackets. The family followed behind. The Tsarina and the girls were all dressed in white and carrying pillows. . . . Yurovsky must have told them to carry pillows to sit on in the automobile. Anna, the Tsarina's maid, came out with *two* pillows.

"Behind her came Dr. Botkin, the cook, the valet," Ermakov recalled. "Nobody seemed excited. I'm sure they didn't suspect."

Orders were given to the driver to start his engine.

Yurovsky then read the death sentence, practically shouting so as to be heard over the roar of the truck engine just outside the door.

"You think the Whites are going to rescue you—but they aren't," Ermakov recalled Yurovsky saying. "You think you're going away to England and be a Tsar again—well, you're not. The Soviet of the Urals sentences you and your family to death for your crimes against the Russian people."

The Tsar seemed not to understand. "What? What?" he shouted back over the roar of the engine. "Aren't we going to get out of here after all?"

"Yurovsky's reply was to fire his pistol straight into the Tsar's face," Ermakov recounted.

"The bullet went right through his brain.

"The Tsar spun to the floor and never moved.

"I fired my Mauser at the Tsarina—only six feet away—couldn't miss. Got her in the mouth. In two seconds she was dead.

"I fired next at Dr. Botkin. He'd thrown up his hands and turned his face half away. The bullet went through his neck. He fell over backwards.

"Yurovsky had shot the Tsarevich out of his chair, and he lay on the floor groaning.

"The cook was crouching in the corner. I got him in the body and then in the head. The valet went down. I don't know who shot him.

"Vaganof made a clean sweep of the girls. They were in a heap on the floor, moaning and dying. He kept pouring bullets into Olga and Tatiana.

"The two younger girls—Maria and Anastasia—had fallen beside Dr. Botkin.

"I don't think any of us hit Anna, the maid. She had slid down in her corner and hidden behind her two pillows. We found afterward that the pillows were crammed with jewels—maybe the jewel cases turned the bullets away. But one of the guards got her through the throat with his bayonet. . . . We had called in our Cheka [secret police] executioners from the corridor to help finish off the job and they were clubbing and bayoneting everybody.

"The Tsarevich wasn't dead . . . still groaning and twisting on the floor. Yurovsky shot him twice more in the head. That finished him.

"Anastasia was still alive too. A guard pushed her over on her back. She shrieked—he beat her to death with his rifle butt."

Ermakov said the dead bodies were then gathered up and put on the truck outside. The room was a shambles: "There was blood everywhere and slippers and pillows and handbags and odds and ends swimming around in a red lake." Ermakov told Halliburton that a total of thirty-eight shots were fired.

It took two hours to cover the twelve miles to the mine. Dawn was breaking by the time the truck arrived. It was too light to burn the bodies by the time they arrived, so Ermakov posted guards around the remains.

During the day of the seventeenth, the Tsar's personal effects were gathered up to be shipped to Moscow.

At 10 P.M. that evening Ermakov was back at the mine. "By the light of the lamps, we stripped the corpses of their clothes. Found a lot of diamonds sewn in the Tsarina's bodice—and more necklaces, gold crosses and a lot of other such things on the girls. These were sent to Moscow along with everything else." The clothes were burned separately. The bodies were taken to the entrance of a mine two kilometers off the highroad.

"Here in the mouth of this mine we built a funeral pyre of cut logs big enough to hold the bodies, two layers deep. We poured five tins of gasoline over the corpses and two buckets of sulphuric acid and set the logs afire. The gasoline made everything burn rapidly. But I stood by to see that not one fingernail or fragment of bone remained unconsumed. Anything of that sort the Whites found I knew they would use as a holy relic. I kept pushing back into the flames whatever pieces were left, and building more fire and pouring on more gasoline. We had to keep the fire burning a long time to burn up the skulls. But I wasn't satisfied till our pyre and everything upon it was reduced to powder."

Ermakov said he collected the ashes, put them in tins and pitched the powdery, imperial remains into the air.

"The wind caught them like dust and carried them out over the woods and fields . . . and it rained the next day . . . so if anybody says he has seen a Romanoff or a piece of a dead one—tell him about the ashes—and the wind—and the rain."

So perished the last Tsar and his family, Ermakov declared: shot by three executioners, their bodies corroded by acid, then burned to powder and scattered over Siberia. I ask the reader's pardon for having quoted this testimony at such length, but it contains several nuggets of truth. Unfortunately these nuggets are buried deep in the rubbish heap of a braggart's lies.

Immediately, one runs up against a contradiction in Ermakov's account. Why bring along *both* sulfuric acid *and* gasoline to destroy the corpses? That is, if the bodies were to be cremated, why bother to disfigure their features with acid first? Clearly the acid would be useful only if the bodies were to be buried, not burned. In itself, this contradiction is not decisive. As I have said earlier in this book, people often do funny, irrational things with bodies. But this contradiction is enough to make us suspicious of Ermakov's reliability as a witness.

Eight days after the murders, White Russian armies under Admiral Alexander Kolchak reconquered Ekaterinburg. The first troops to reach the Ipatiev house found a chaos of broken furniture, empty rooms and debris. The semibasement room where the executions had taken place looked freshly scrubbed, but there were bullet holes and bayonet gouges in the walls.

Rumors led the White Army investigators to an abandoned mine, twelve feet deep, about twelve miles outside the city at a place called Koptyaki, near four lonely pine trees named "The Four Brothers."

In and around the mine shaft a total of sixty-five half-combusted relics were found amid the ashes of two bonfires. Among them were what army investigators concluded were the Tsar's belt buckle, the Tsarevich's belt buckle, an emerald cross, topaz beads, a pearl earring, an Ulm Cross (a tsarist military decoration), an eyeglass lens, three small icons, the Empress's spectacles case, buttons and hooks that seemed to belong to women's corsets, fragments of military caps worn by Nicholas and Alexei, shoe buckles belonging to the Grand Duchesses, and Dr. Botkin's upper denture plate.

A single, severed human finger belonging to a middle-aged woman was also found. It was the sole human fragment unearthed. The remains of a small dog were also found.

The White Army was driven back from Ekaterinburg, but eventually the results of the investigations were assembled and published. The investigators were not able to solve the riddle of the missing corpses.

Ekaterinburg was renamed Sverdlovsk, after Yakov Sverdlov, the member of the Bolshevik Central Committee who ordered the executions from Moscow, almost certainly with Lenin's approval. Sverdlovsk itself became a munitions manufacturing city, off limits to all foreigners and to most Russian citizens. Soviet T-31 tanks were built there during World War II. American U-2 pilot Francis Gary Powers was shot down over Sverdlovsk in 1962 while attempting to photograph its military secrets.

Subsequent political crosscurrents in Russia further obscure the story. Some of the participants in the slaughter were supporters of Josef Stalin's rival, Leon Trotsky. After Trotsky's purge and assassination, these protagonists in the Tsar's murder officially ceased to exist. Everything they did, including their role in killing the Tsar, was blotted out from Soviet history books.

By 1935 the Ipatiev house, where the shootings had taken place, was a museum celebrating the death of the "crowned hangman," as Nicholas was called by the Bolsheviks. Halliburton toured it and saw excerpts from the Tsar's diaries on display there. By 1959, however, the house had become a state archive, off limits to the public. In

1977 it was bulldozed, because local Communist authorities were alarmed that the house was gradually becoming a goal of pilgrims from all over Russia, who were coming here to pay homage to the memory of the Tsar. Our hosts told us that the local Communist Party boss who ordered its destruction was none other than Boris Yeltsin, who has since risen to the very pinnacle of power in the Russian government. Today he is President of Russia.

In the decades that passed, a cloak of silence descended over the murders. Initially extolled as an act of revolutionary justice, the wholesale massacre of the Tsar and his family horrified the rest of the world and gradually became an embarrassment to the new Soviet regime. As the newspaper headline quoted earlier attests, the Bolsheviks never spoke of the fate of the Tsar's family and entourage, only of the Tsar's execution. People began to wonder if, by some miracle or mischance, some or even all of the Tsar's family might have survived the bloodbath at the Ipatiev house. This official silence, complicated by subsequent contradictions, has given rise to a host of claimants to the crown of the Romanovs. There have been multiple Anastasias, nearly as many Alexeis, no shortage of Alexandras, Olgas, Tatianas and Maries. Some even insist the Tsar himself escaped his firing squad and left the country to live quietly in Poland. I myself receive letters from time to time, from a woman who lives in a trailer park in Hialeah, near Miami, who believes herself to be Anastasia. She illustrates the letters with weird ideograms: weeping eyes, shining crucifixes, mysterious question marks. The Romanovs cast a long shadow, even today.

The most famous of these claimants was a woman who surfaced in 1920 in Berlin after a suicide attempt. The woman had total amnesia but bore a striking resemblance to Anastasia, the Tsar's youngest daughter. She could not speak Russian but seemed to recall remarkable details of court protocol and Romanov family history, enough to convince some people that she was truly Anastasia. Known as Anna Anderson, this woman spent her whole life trying to prove her identity. She died in 1984 in Virginia, aged eighty-two, and her remains were cremated. Locks of her cut hair survive but, as we shall see, these may be of doubtful value in weighing her claim to royal blood.

In the 1980s the Soviet Union embarked on a new period of "openness" and "restructuring" advocated by the new President and Communist Party chairman, Mikhail Gorbachev. Suddenly thousands of secret documents were declassified.

A Soviet playwright, Edvard Radzinsky, had been quietly researching the death of the Tsar for nearly twenty-five years. When the archives of Moscow's Museum of the October Revolution were finally opened to scholars in the late 1980s, Radzinsky found a treasure trove of old receipts, diaries and dossiers, including the fifty-volume diary of Tsar Nicholas II himself, and signed eyewitness reports written by his assassins, Yurovsky and Ermakov. There was even a 1964 tape recording by Grigori Nikulin, Yurovsky's lieutenant, who participated in the killings.

The most important of these documents was the so-called "Yurovsky Note," an after-action report written by the chief assassin, in which he refers to himself as "the commandant." Gradually a fairly complete picture of the murders emerged. It was a brutal tale of blood, deceit, boasting, drunkenness and ghoulish bungling. A synopsis is contained in Radzinsky's 1992 book, *The Last Tsar*.

According to the Yurovsky Note, twelve men were in the firing squad: six unidentified Latvian guards, Yurovsky, Ermakov, Yurovsky's right-hand man Grigori Nikulin and a deserter from the Tsar's Life Guards named Alexei Kabanov, as well as two secret policemen named Pavel Medvedev and Mikhail Medvedev-Kudrin.

The royal family had gone to bed at 10:30 P.M. Shortly before midnight they were awakened and told to go downstairs. Ostensibly they were being transferred to a jail nearer the center of the city, which was besieged by White Russian armies.

Once assembled in the semibasement room at the rear of the house, the Tsar and his entourage were arranged in two rows. They were persuaded to group themselves quietly by means of a simple ruse: Yurovsky told them they were going to have their pictures taken in order to disprove rumors that they were dead. Obediently,

Nicholas and the others took their places. To lend credence to this cruel hoax, two chairs were brought in: one for the invalid heir Alexei, the other for the Tsarina.

Outside the Fiat truck engine roared to life, creating an unholy din. Yurovsky read out a decree from the Ural Soviet condemning the Tsar and his family to death. The noise from the truck was so loud that Nicholas could not hear what Yurovsky was saying. "What? What?" the Tsar asked. Yurovsky read the decree again, but before he was finished the shooting began. The Tsar's last words may have been: "Forgive them, for they know not what they do." Yurovsky, Ermakov and Medvedev would later dispute who shot the Tsar first. Years later all three men sent their pistols to the Museum of the Revolution in Moscow, each claiming his was the weapon that had slain the Tsar.

A double door leading to an adjacent room crashed open and the six Latvian guards poured their gunfire into the room. The assassins stood so close together that they gave each other powder burns as they jostled and fired into the screaming royal family. But a macabre situation developed. Though Nicholas had died instantly, certain others of the victims proved harder to kill. Bullets were actually ricocheting off their bodies, spanging into the walls of the room.

"Alexei, three of his sisters, the lady-in-waiting and Botkin were still alive. They had to be finished off," Yurovsky wrote in his after-action report. "This amazed the commandant since we had aimed straight for the heart. It was also surprising that the bullets from the revolvers bounced off for some reason and ricocheted, jumping around the room like hail."

Yurovsky was puzzled by the "strange vitality" of Alexei and gave him the coup de grâce by firing two revolver shots into his head at close range. But the women proved even harder to kill. After exhausting their magazines, the Latvian guards rushed forward and used their bayonets to finish the grisly job. But even these rough-and-ready weapons seemed to turn aside against the chests and torsos of the women.

Only later was it discovered that the corsets the women were wearing were stuffed with diamonds and precious stones. These acted as bulletproof vests and prolonged their owners' agony. Yurovsky wrote that, when the corpses were stripped later, eighteen pounds of diamonds were recovered from the corsets.

The bodies were then loaded onto the truck and driven to the Four Brothers Mine, twelve miles away, near the village of Koptyaki. There they were stripped naked and their clothing was rummaged through and burned. Nikulin was later given the errand of taking the jewels to Moscow. The corpses were dumped into the mine shaft, which was only about eight feet deep, and hand grenades were flung in and exploded after them to seal the hole.

(This would explain the sixty-five charred, scattered relics found by the White Russian investigators when they later searched the area near the Four Brothers Mine. The single human finger had apparently been blown off a hand of one of the women by the hand grenade explosions and was overlooked by the assassins later.)

But the story did not end here. To his disgust and chagrin, Yurovsky found that the whereabouts of the "secret" burial site were the talk of the town. The flamboyant Ermakov, who had apparently been drunk throughout the assassinations, had enlisted a band of equally drunken assistants to help with the disposal of the bodies, and these had later boasted of their deeds.

Now, with the White Russian armies closing in, Yurovsky and his followers had to bury the Tsar and his family all over again. The next night, with torches, ropes, kerosene and sulfuric acid, Yurovsky returned to the death pit at the Four Brothers Mine, determined to dispose of the telltale corpses for good. A Bolshevik sailor named Vaganov, the "Vaganof" of Ermakov's account, was sent into the muddy hole to knot ropes around the bodies, which were then hauled up.

The muddy, mutilated bodies were loaded aboard carts, but these proved too rickety to be serviceable. Yurovsky then sent back to town for a truck. Daylight came and went. At nightfall on the nineteenth, nearly three days after the murders, Yurovsky and his band set out with the hideous, bloated, flyblown remains of "The

Autocrat of All the Russias," as Nicholas II was known in life, his wife, his children and his servants.

It had been a rainy summer and the truck kept getting stuck in the mud. Yurovsky and his helpers put planks under the wheels over and over again, but by 4:30 A.M. the truck slipped into a bog so deep it could not be moved.

There was no more time. The bodies would have to be disposed of on the spot. Yurovsky burned two of them: Alexei and a female who he at first thought was the Tsarina Alexandra but later decided must have been her maid, Anna Demidova. This confusion on Yurovsky's part as to the identity of the female would lend hope to those who believed Anastasia had somehow escaped the slaughter. At any rate, Yurovsky seems to have badly underestimated the amount of time needed to combust fully a human corpse—it is an error many murderers make. He may also have run out of fuel.

Exhausted, disgusted, all out of time, with dawn breaking, the commandant ordered a pit dug six feet deep and eight feet square. In it, in the midst of a random stretch of bog, near a railroad crossing, the Tsar and the rest of his entourage were flung and hastily buried. The hole was so shallow that Yurovsky worried that the corpse stench would rise through the earth. He decided to kill the smell with sulfuric acid.

"The bodies were doused with sulfuric acid so they couldn't be recognized and to prevent any stink from them rotting. We scattered it with dirt and lime, put boards on top, and rode over it several times—no trace of the hole remained. The secret was kept—the Whites did not find this burial site," Yurovsky wrote in his report.

Throughout the 1980s, Radzinsky published several articles in a Soviet periodical about his inquiries into the death of the Tsar. He received thousands of letters in response, many of them from people who remembered other details, or who knew the assassins personally.

Then, in April 1989, the final breakthrough came: a Soviet mystery writer named Geli Ryabov described in the avant-garde weekly, *Moscow News*, how he and Dr. Alexander Avdonin, an Ekaterinburg geophysicist, had located the skeletons of the Tsar and his family in a shallow grave outside Sverdlovsk in 1979. Not daring to reveal his discovery, Ryabov had waited a decade to make it public.

My colleagues and I first heard of the discovery in 1992, at a convention of the American Academy of Forensic Sciences in New Orleans. We saw press reports about the discovery of the bodies, and in these it was said that the U. S. Secretary of State, James Baker, had been shown the remains on a visit to Ekaterinburg. The Russians had asked Baker if the United States might provide technical assistance in identifying them.

The mystery of the Romanovs had fascinated me for more than four decades. This was a unique opportunity to shine the light of modern science into the dark recesses of one of the most baffling and enigmatic mass murders in this century. Few deaths had been so momentous and mysterious as that of the Tsar and his household. Seventy years of Soviet history had played out since that midnight in Ekaterinburg, yet the final fate of the Romanovs remained as great a riddle as ever. The corpse of Lenin had been preserved under glass in Red Square. Had the bones of the Tsar been preserved under peat and mud in a Northeast Asian bog? I immediately bent my thoughts toward Russia.

While still in New Orleans, I asked the armed forces medical examiner if he had received any official request to help the Russians. I didn't want to intrude on someone else's investigation. He told me he had heard nothing of this case; therefore his department was not involved with the Romanovs at all. So the way was clear.

I immediately organized an extremely impressive team of experts. Besides myself, there was Dr. Lowell Levine; Dr. Michael Baden; Cathryn Oakes, a hair and fiber microscopist with the New York State Police Department who has since become Mrs. Levine; my wife Margaret, a media specialist who would assist us in documenting and videotaping the investigation; and William Goza, a retired Gainesville attorney and historian, who is president of several foundations and possesses formidable diplomatic skills. On two later trips to Ekaterinburg we were fortunate to have the help of two outstanding Florida medical examiners, Dr. William Hamilton and Dr. Alexander Melamud. Dr. Melamud speaks Russian like a native —as well he should, for he was born and raised in the Ukraine.

What finally opened the door for us was a fax from the president of the University of Florida, Dr. John Lombardi, to Dr. Alexander Avdonin, the Soviet geophysicist who had personally helped unearth the remains. Some weeks passed. Finally we received an official invitation jointly signed by Dr. Avdonin and Dr. Alexander Blokhin, vice-president for the public health district of Sverdlovsk. We packed our bags and flew to Russia.

We were met at the airport at Ekaterinburg by Dr. Avdonin and Dr. Nikolai Nevolin, who heads the state forensic bureau for the district of Sverdlovsk. The remains were entrusted to his care and were kept at his institute. The very next morning we were permitted to see them.

At last the final door swung open and we were let into the room containing the rediscovered bones. Immediately we faced a procedural obstacle. The Russians initially refused to let us photograph the remains. This was a bitter blow, and we objected strenuously. All our work would be in vain if we were not able to document our findings. On their side, the Russians were understandably worried that we would steal their thunder and make commercial capital out of some of the most extraordinary human skeletons ever found.

We reached a temporary compromise. We would examine the remains for several hours, without cameras, that morning. Later we would renew our request to take photographs. I had the feeling that the Russians were sizing us up, trying to tell if we were true experts or just glib dilettantes.

I was able to set them straight within the next few hours. By the end of the morning I managed, on the basis of the unlabeled skeletal remains before me, to decide the age and sex of all the skeletons and to assign them tentative identifications. The speed and accuracy of my initial analysis produced a gratifying response: suddenly, the Russians were looking at us with unfeigned respect. They had taken months to make their identifications, using numerous experts in various fields, working independently. We had arrived at roughly the same conclusions in a few hours. I told our hosts we could go no further unless we could document what we were doing. We went to lunch while discussions were held about our photographic access. When we got back from lunch, all barriers had been removed. Now we could begin our examination in earnest.

The nine skeletons were identified only by number. Five were female, four male. Of the five females, three were young women, only recently grown to maturity. All the faces were badly fractured, every single one. This fact made reconstruction of facial features risky or impossible, but it also conformed to the accounts of the assassinations: that the faces of the victims were smashed in with rifle butts to render them unrecognizable.

All of the female skeletons had dental work. None of the males did, though we knew from historical records that Dr. Botkin had a denture plate in his upper jaw, which was later extricated from the mud of the Four Brothers Mine by the White Army investigators. Sure enough, one of the males had a few teeth in his lower jaw, no teeth at all in his upper jaw, and probably wore false teeth in life.

The enamel surfaces of the teeth showed the signs of acid etching. The outer tables of the cranial vaults were eroded away by acid also. A single broken jar that had once contained sulfuric acid was also found among the remains. This, too, agreed with accounts of the killings. A receipt for 400 pounds of sulfuric acid, requisitioned shortly before the murders, still exists in Russian archives. I have seen copies of this receipt with my own eyes.

In all, fourteen bullets were recovered from the grave, along with the remains of one hand grenade detonator. All the bullets were 7.62, 7.63 or 7.65mm, about the equivalent of .32-caliber bullets. The Russians told us they believed nine of the bullets came from Nagants, four came possibly from a Browning and one from some other gun, possibly a Mauser. These bullets had almost certainly lodged in the bodies at the time of death, but twelve of them had gradually come loose as the remains decomposed. The Russians told us that loose teeth had also been found in the shallow grave, mixed in among the bones.

Three bodies, Numbers 2, 3 and 6, had through-and-through gunshot wounds to the head. Another body, No. 9, had a stab wound in the breastbone that could have been made by a bayonet. It is important to remember that not every lethal wound, whether it be a bullet or a knife thrust, will leave a mark on the skeleton under-neath, even when the ribs and vertebrae are recovered intact, which was certainly not the case here.

· Body No. 1 was identified by its pelvis as a fully grown female. The skull was missing its facial bones. There was a gold bridge of poor workmanship on the mandible—not very expensive dental work. But the most revealing detail turned up in my examination of the ankle joints. These showed an extension of the joint surfaces, as if the woman had spent many hours crouching or kneeling, perhaps while she was scrubbing floors or doing other menial work. On the basis of these joints, together with the overall composition of the group, I believe this skeleton belonged to the Tsarina's maid, Anna Demidova.

· Body No. 2, alone among the remains, still had its torso intact, held together by adipocere, a grayish-white waxy substance that forms when fatty tissue combine with water after death. It was first noticed and mentioned by Sir Thomas Browne, the seventeenth-century es-sayist, whose description remains classically true today:

> Teeth, bones, and hair, give the most lasting defiance to corruption. In an Hydropicall body ten years buried in a Church-yard, we met with a fat concretion, where the nitre of the Earth, and salt and lixivious liquor of the body, had coagulated large lumps of fat, into the consistence of the hardest castle-soap.

From the adipocere in this body the Russians had recovered one bullet in the pelvic area and one from a vertebra.

The skeleton belonged to a mature man with a very flat, sloping forehead. I believe it is that of Dr. Sergei Botkin, the physician who watched over the young Tsarevich Alexei, who died with the family, and whose photograph in life closely matched the shape of this forehead. The skull had no upper teeth, and Botkin's dental plate had been found by White Russian investigators over seventy years earlier at the mouth of the Four Brothers Mine. The skull had a gunshot wound from a bullet that entered the left frontal bone in the upper left corner of the forehead and exited through the right temporal area.

In 1935, Ermakov told Halliburton that Dr. Botkin "had thrown up his hands and turned his face half away." Though Ermakov erroneously reported that he believed Botkin was shot in the throat, the detail of the doctor partly turning his head away squared very well with the skull of Body No. 2.

· Body No. 3's skeleton belonged to a young adult female with a bulging forehead, in her early twenties when she died. It has been tentatively identified as belonging to the young Grand Duchess Olga. The shape of the head agrees extraordinarily closely with lifetime photographs of Olga. Half of her middle face, the facial bones between the tops of the eye orbits and the lower jaw, was missing. She clearly was completely grown, and the roots of her third molars, her "wisdom teeth," were fully developed. Regrettably the bones of the legs were not intact; they had been cut into sections after being dug up but before we arrived on the scene. As a result, they could not be used for height estimates. Instead we used bones from the arms to estimate the female's height. Though arm lengths are not as reliable as leg lengths, we arrived at a height estimate of 64.9 inches. Dr. Levine found extensive amalgam fillings in her teeth, a trait shared by the other two young females. It is very likely they were fond of sweets, in life.

In Body No. 3, the bullet entered under the left jaw, broke the jaw, went through the palate behind the nose and exited through the frontal bone of the skull. Such a trajectory could come from a gun placed under the chin and fired up, or from firing at a body already lying on the floor. The exit wound was very neat, drilled in a near-perfect circle. The top of the skull showed signs of acid etching.

I will pass over Body No. 4 for now, and return to it later, for reasons that will become apparent.

· Body No. 5 belonged to a woman in her late teens or early twenties. Half of her middle face was missing, a pattern of damage already seen in Body No. 3. Dr. Levine and I agreed that she was the youngest of the five women whose skeletons lay before us. We concluded this from the fact that the root tips of her third molars were incomplete. Her sacrum, in the back of her pelvis, was not completely developed. Her limb bones showed that growth had only recently ended. Her back showed evidence of immaturity, but it was nevertheless the back of a woman at least eighteen years old. We estimated her height at 67.5 inches. The Russians told us that a bullet had been found in a lump of adipocere near this body. We believe this skeleton is that of Marie, who was nineteen years old at the time of the murders.

· Body No. 6 belonged to a young woman who was nevertheless fully grown. Her dental and skeletal development fell neatly between that of Bodies 3 and 5. There was no evidence of recent growth in her limb bones. Her sacrum and pelvic rim were mature, which made her at least eighteen. On the basis of her limb bones, we put her height at 65.6 inches, right between the other two young females. More important, her collarbone was mature, making her at least twenty years old. The Grand Duchess Tatiana was twenty-one years and two months old at the time of the shootings, so this skeleton agreed very closely with the historical record.

Body No. 6 had a gunshot entrance wound high on the back left side of the skull, and an associated exit wound just in front of the right temple. The minimum diameter of the entrance wound was 8.8mm, which would be consistent with the .32-caliber handguns used in the assassinations. A slug from a .32 is 7.6mm in diameter. This young woman had been shot in the back of the head.

So: 3, 5 and 6 were Olga, Marie and Tatiana, in that order. Where was Anastasia? None of these three young female skeletons was young enough to be Anastasia, who was seventeen years and one month old the night of the shootings. Our Russian hosts believed that Body No. 6, the midmost of the three young females, was the long-lost Anastasia. Alas! We had to disagree, based on the growth patterns of the teeth, pelvises, sacra and long limbs of the three skeletons before us. The Russians had labored manfully over Body No. 6, attempting to restore its facial bones with generous dollops of glue, stretched across wide gaps. They had been forced to estimate over and over again, while reassembling these fragments, almost none of which were touching each other in the reconstruction. It was a remarkable and ingenious exercise, but it was too fanciful for me to buy: Anastasia was not in this room.

Another piece of evidence was the height of the skeletal remains. This young woman was roughly the same height as the other two young women whose remains were discovered in the mass grave. In photographs of Anastasia taken with her sisters a year before her death, she is shorter than Olga and noticeably shorter than Tatiana and Marie.

There are no photographs of the royal family in the months immediately preceding the shootings. Could Anastasia have undergone a "growth spurt" in those months before the shootings? Could she have suddenly "caught up" with her sisters in stature? It is extremely unlikely.

In September 1917, only ten months before the shootings, while she was under house arrest in Tobolsk, the Tsarina Alexandra wrote in her diary: "Anastasia is very fat, like Marie used to be—big, thick-waisted, then tiny feet—*I hope she grows more. . . .*" (My italics.) Though the quote is rather vague, it seems to indicate clearly that Anastasia was not yet as tall as her sisters, and might be expected to grow taller.

I will pass over Body No. 7 for the moment, and return to it presently.

· The skeleton of Body No. 8 was very fragmentary and was grievously damaged by acid. It belonged to an adult male in his forties or fifties. The maxilla (upper jaw) of Body No. 8 was not recovered. The mandible was recovered, but it had lost its remaining teeth at death. The area immediately above the eye orbits, where our eyebrows are in life, was noticeably flat. The owner of this skull, when alive, had a flattened profile. From the hip and pelvic remains, this skeleton was clearly male. He does not appear to have been very big. One ulna was fractured and later healed. I believe this to have been the skeleton of the cook, Ivan Mikhailovich Kharitonov, mainly by a process of elimination that I will explain later.

· The skeleton of Body No. 9 belonged to a big, heavy-boned man over six feet tall, who was beginning to show evidence of aging. The back of the skull was missing. The teeth were worn. There was a stab wound, probably by a bayonet, through the breastbone from front to back, but I am convinced this particular breastbone does not belong to this set of remains. For the rest, the robust size of the skeleton agrees well with descriptions we have of the footman, Alexei Igorevich Trupp, who was part of the Tsar's entourage at Ekaterinburg.

We have now discussed Bodies 1, 2, 3, 5, 6, 8 and 9. Let us return to Bodies 4 and 7, in reverse order.

· Body No. 7 was in some ways the most important of all that were found in the pit. It belonged to an older woman whose rib cage may have been damaged by bayonet thrusts—the bones were not well enough preserved to allow me to say this with certainty. But it was not these that commanded our attention. Rather, it was her amazing and exquisite dental work. My colleague, Dr. Levine, initially thought the two silvery crowns in the lower jaw were aluminum "temporaries." They weren't. To his astonishment, he found they were made of platinum. When we took flash pictures of this skull, the gleaming platinum crowns coruscated brilliantly in the sudden light. Dr. Levine also discovered beautiful porcelain crowns in this skull's jaws, along with wonderfully wrought gold fillings. It was stunning dental work, extremely costly and cunningly contrived.

It was this rich dental work, so precious-metaled it was far beyond the means of all but the richest Russians, that convinced the men who initially excavated the mass grave that here, at last, were the remains of the royal family. The Tsarina Alexandra mentions visiting the dentist several times in her diaries, and it is well that she did. The Bolshevik assassins despoiled the Tsarina of her jewels, but they could not take her teeth; and these beautiful tooth crowns spoke eloquently even in death. Taken together with the scattered bullets, the bits of rope and the smashed jar of sulfuric acid, these teeth were a powerful signal to the excavators that they were dealing with the grave of the Tsar and his family.

· Body No. 4 I believe to be the skeleton of Tsar Nicholas II. It belonged to a middle-aged man of fairly short stature. The skeleton possessed a clearly male pelvis. The skull had a very broad, flat palate that is consistent with the mouth shape of the Tsar in photographs taken before he grew his beard. It had a jutting brow line, and so did the Tsar: the curving, protruding supraorbital bones are consistent with photographs of Nicholas taken during his life. The hipbones showed the characteristic wear and deformation produced by many hours on horseback, and we know the Tsar was an ardent horseman.

The only jarring note was struck by the extraordinary, rotten condition of this skeleton's teeth, and the complete absence of dental work. There was not a single filling in any of the remaining teeth. All these were worn to gray nubbins. The lower jaw showed clear inroads of periodontal disease. The owner of these teeth was long overdue for dentures. Why didn't he get them? As Tsar, he could surely afford a good dentist!

I believe Nicholas must have had a horror of dentists and, because he was Tsar, no one could force him to visit one. Rank has its privileges, and among them is the liberty to let your teeth go to rack and ruin if you desire. Was the Tsar a coward before the dentist's drill? Did he have a horror of physical pain? His jaws seemed to say so. Is it speculating too far, to glimpse in these rotten, neglected teeth a vivid, concrete symbol of the Russian royal family in those final years, falling to pieces, but nevertheless unwilling to take the necessary, painful steps needed to repair the damage and save themselves? Perhaps, perhaps not.

I picked up the skull and held it in my hands, staring at it intently. It was a gray thing with a crushed face. A dark void yawned in the middle of its features, below the eye sockets and above the jaw. Blows of terrific force had shattered its features. I was haunted by the line in George Orwell's *Nineteen Eighty-Four*, a nightmarish view of the future based partly on the already famous brutality of the Soviet state: *"If you want a picture of the future, imagine a boot stamping on a human face—forever. . . ."* The Tsar's skull was grievously mutilated, the remains perfectly consistent with his fate. He was among the first, and certainly the foremost, victims of Bolshevik savagery.

Yet he had endured. Even his bad teeth had outlasted the outlaw state that had slain him, then tried to hide him away forever in the nameless darkness of an unmarked pit. Now Nicholas II, onetime Tsar of All the Russias, had risen back up into the light of day, accompanied by most of his family and a handful of his servants.

As I mused on these ironies, an eerie thing happened. We were passing the skull around among ourselves, when we heard something dully rattling inside the braincase. Training a flashlight on the base of the skull, peering in through the aperture where the spinal cord would have been anchored, we descried a small, dried, shrunken object about the size of a small pear, rolling to and fro. It was the desiccated brain of Tsar Nicholas II.

For I am quite convinced this was the Tsar's skull. None of the other three male skeletons came so close to the profile of Nicholas II in life as did this set of remains. No. 2, Dr. Botkin, had a very distinct, flat, sloping forehead and wore dentures, as we know Botkin did in life. No. 9 was far too tall and too old to be the Tsar. It was almost certainly Trupp, the sixty-one-year-old footman. No. 8, the most fragmentary of the male skeletons, had been heavily doused with acid and it was initially thought that these remains had been singled out for special disfigurement, perhaps as a sign of rank. But the features of the skull in no way agree with the countenance of the

Tsar in life, especially in the unpronounced brow line. These are the remains of Kharitonov, the cook. They were more damaged by acid, not because of any especial spite, but because they lay deepest in the pit, at the very bottom.

Indeed, the more we studied the demography of the group, the more we were struck by the congruence of the skeletons with the stories of the execution of the Tsar and his family. All the skeletons propped each other up. Each contributed to the authenticity of the other. In the end, the ensemble formed a powerful web of circumstantial evidence, reinforced from within by skeletal remains of extraordinary singularity. Consider these points:

There is one skeleton to fit everyone known to be in the party, with the exception of the Tsarevich Alexei and Anastasia, who are missing. If you were to go out at random and try to assemble such a group, to fit such historical descriptions, you would have to be remarkably lucky or do incredible physical examinations to make sure everything fits. At the time of the shootings, the Tsar was fifty, the Tsarina Alexandra forty-six. Olga was twenty-two years and nine months old; Tatiana had just turned twenty-one; Marie's nineteenth birthday had just come five weeks before; and Anastasia was seventeen years and one month old. Alexei was just two weeks short of his fourteenth birthday. The maid Demidova was forty. The footman, Trupp, was sixty-one and the cook, Kharitonov, was forty-eight.

When we compare these ages, and the other things we know of the royal family and their entourage, with the evidence of the skeletons, everything aligns nicely. Demidova's skeleton is of the right age and sex. Botkin's skeleton has the right forehead, the right age, the right sex, the right dental information. The three young women's skeletons, as well as that of the oldest woman, have features in common that are often seen in families, suggesting they were related. The three young women all have the same type of dental work in their mouths, suggesting they all were treated by the same dentist. The remaining older woman's skeleton shares these same features, so she is related to them. The oldest woman has the exceptional rich dental work which is confirmed from numerous mentions in Alexandra's diaries. The Tsar's skeleton is the right age, the right height, with the right facial features. The skeleton of the footman, Trupp, shows the worn teeth and age and sex and height we would expect. That of the cook, Kharitonov, also displays the right age and sex.

Everything about the burial suggests urgent haste and the need for secrecy, which agrees very well with the historical circumstances. Remember, White Russian armies were closing in on Ekaterinburg in those days. The faces are bludgeoned to render them unrecognizable, just in case they are found. Sulfuric acid is flung over them, to complete the disfigurement. The corpses are buried in an unmarked grave, together with the ropes used to haul them and the jar of acid used to disfigure them. We know from Ermakov that .32-caliber weapons were used, and sure enough, .32-caliber bullets are later recovered from the grave. The receipt for the sulfuric acid is a matter of record. Everything fits.

Or almost everything. None of the nine skeletons could be attributed to the fourteen-year-old Tsarevich Alexei, and none of them, despite the Russians' initial hopes, could be identified with a girl seventeen years and one month old: Anastasia.

In his confidential after-action report, Yurovsky described burning two bodies beside the pit. One was that of the Tsarevich. The other belonged to a female, who he at first thought was the Tsarina Alexandra, but later decided must have been the maid, Demidova.

This confusion has given one last straw to grasp at to the resurrectionists who believe Anastasia escaped the hecatomb that engulfed her family. How, these stubborn optimists ask, would it be possible for Yurovsky to confuse the corpse of a seventeen-year-old girl with that of two other women, one of them forty years old, the other fifty? Was "Anna Anderson," who died an old woman in 1984, telling the truth? Was she the last of the Romanovs?

I very much doubt it. I believe I can explain why Yurovsky mixed up the female corpses. My long experience with decayed human remains has given me a weary familiarity with the quirks of dissolution.

Remember, the Tsar and his party were killed in summertime, in

July 1918, in warm weather. Blood would have soaked the disheveled hair of the victims, which would have then dried into a dark hard mass. The bodies had decomposed for three days in daytime temperatures averaging roughly 70 degrees Fahrenheit. Bloating would be pronounced, and bloating makes it very difficult to guess the original weight or girth of a set of remains.

Furthermore you must remember that all of the bodies, except perhaps for that of Alexei, the son, were reportedly stripped of all clothing. Clothing would have been an easy means of telling the bodies apart, and now that indicator was gone. All in all, the nude and bloated torsos of the females would have taken on a remarkable, balloonish anonymity.

Next, flies must be considered. Flies lay their eggs during the first daylight hours in which they can reach a dead body. Those eggs begin to hatch a couple of days later in a sudden burst of activity. There were plenty of flies in that area—I observed them myself, during my visit. These bodies had many wounds. Their faces had been smashed to bloody pulp. They were left in the open near the shaft of the Four Brothers Mine all day long after the executions, then thrown into a mine shaft and hand grenades were flung down on them, further mangling the remains. Flies would have had ample opportunity to lay eggs on the eyes, nostrils and other apertures, along with the open wounds. These eggs and the resulting maggots, deposited in a thick, foamy froth over the mutilated faces, would have further masked the bodies' identities.

Then, when word got out that the bodies were at the Four Brothers Mine, Yurovsky and his henchmen had to exhume the bodies and rebury them somewhere else. In all, three days passed between the time of the shootings and the final burial in the unmarked pit.

The bloating, the hard, blood-soaked hair of the women, the absence of clothing and the encrustation of fly eggs and maggots on their faces, the enveloping darkness—all these factors would have rendered the remains very hard to identify. It would be quite possible to mistake one female for another.

At any rate this is what I believe happened. Yurovsky burned two bodies, as he reported. One belonged to the young Tsarevich Alexei; the other was Anastasia. This explains why the skeletons of the two youngest children were not among those on the tables at the forensic bureau.

Is it even remotely possible that Anastasia and Alexei survived? Is it conceivable that some kindhearted Bolshevik spirited them away? Is it thinkable that, despite their wounds, wounds that would have been doubly injurious to a hemophiliac like Alexei, the missing royal children lived, recovered their health and escaped to the West? Of course it is. I merely say it is highly unlikely. My experience with murder, ancient and modern, makes it hard for me to believe in these far-fetched mercies.

In 1964, Grigori Nikulin, Yurovsky's assistant during the killings, was persuaded to make a tape of his reminiscences of the event. By this time most of the original assassins were dead. Yurovsky himself died a painful death from an ulcer in 1938. The flamboyant Ermakov, who gave his "deathbed" interview to Halliburton in 1935, outlived the young journalist by years, dying only in 1952 after recounting his exploits over and over again to young Soviet Pioneers gathered around campfires.

Nikulin was a sober, cold-blooded young killer at the time of the assassinations. Yurovsky had recruited him personally and was extremely fond of him, even calling him his "son." Nikulin moreover was a teetotaler. His account of the evening therefore carried far more weight than the lurid account of the drunken, lying Ermakov.

Persuaded with great difficulty to come to the radio studio in 1964, Nikulin nonetheless stubbornly refused to discuss details of the murders.

"There's no need to savor it. Let it remain with us. Let it depart with us," he said tersely.

Asked about the tale of the "Anastasia" who had somehow dodged the bullets and escaped to the West, Nikulin replied briefly, in the flat, simple diction of one who knew.

"They all perished," he said.

In 1993 there was a dramatic new development in the story of the royal bones. DNA tests carried out in Great Britain have matched a blood sample from the British royal family with the DNA recovered from the Russian skeletons, with a 98.5 percent degree of certainty. Dr. Mary-Claire King at the University of California, Berkeley, has worked on samples we brought back and has confirmed what the British had reported.

DNA (deoxyribonucleic acid) is the substance that contains the genetic code that makes each human being unique. There are two types of DNA present in each living cell, nuclear DNA and mitochondrial DNA. The first type, called nuclear or genomic DNA, is quickly lost during heating or decomposition in human remains. It will linger longer in a dried sample of blood, or semen on clothing; but by the time human remains have begun to decompose, it is virtually impossible to isolate nuclear DNA anymore. Bacteria swarm in the remains, flies move in and pollute the body with their DNA, and what is left is a messy hodgepodge that is useless for nuclear DNA sampling.

Fortunately, the second type of DNA, mitochondrial DNA, lies not in the nucleus but outside, in the cell itself. This substance is present in the female ovum and in the tail of the male sperm, but when the sperm fertilizes the egg at the moment of conception, the tail of the sperm breaks off. Thus the mitochondrial DNA of the male is lost, and only that of the female is passed on to each of the offspring. And it is passed on without variation, from one generation to the next. Every single child has the mitochondrial DNA of its mother, who has the mitochondrial DNA of her mother, and so on. Changes in mitochondrial DNA are extremely rare, and happen on the order of once every three to four thousand years. That is the wonderful thing about mitochondrial DNA. It stays the same in a family for generation after generation and is passed on through the female line. It can endure in our bones for hundreds of years, if they are not cremated.

In the case of the Romanovs, we can easily go back to Queen

Victoria, who has been described as the grandmother of Europe's royal families. Queen Victoria, like any mother, passed her mitochondrial DNA on to her offspring. And one of her daughters passed that same mitochondrial DNA on to her offspring, one of whom was Alexandra, the wife of Tsar Nicholas II. And Alexandra passed her mitochondrial DNA on to all her children. Similarly Alexandra's sister, Princess Victoria of Hesse, passed it on to her children, one of whom was the mother of Prince Philip, the Duke of Edinburgh, and his sisters. Therefore the mitochondrial DNA found in the blood of Prince Philip would be identical to that of Queen Victoria and the Tsarina Alexandra. It only remained to carry out the necessary tests.

These were performed in July 1993 near London. Prince Philip submitted a sample of his blood and its DNA was extracted. At the same time, Pavel Ivanov, head of the DNA unit at the Russian Academy of Sciences, brought a sample of the Romanov bones to Great Britain. There, using a technique called PCR or polymerase chain reaction, a small sample of DNA was extracted from the bones and grown in a culture.

There are only four nucleotides that make up all mitochondrial DNA: cytosine, adenine, thymine and guanine, known as CATG for short. In mitochondrial DNA there are 16,569 base pairs of nucleotides, arranged in a ring. A computer printout of a DNA sequence looks like a diabolically complex code, based on just four letters in neat columns, repeated again and again in slightly varying order for page after page. Luckily we do not have to scrutinize all 16,569 pairs. We can focus on certain "hyper-variable regions," made up of a total of just 608 base pairs. Computers are of great help in matching up the hyper-variable regions. When the results for the hyper-variable regions in two DNA samples match up at these crucial checkpoints, you can be virtually certain they are the same.

This is what happened when Prince Philip's blood DNA was matched up with the Romanovs' bone DNA. Dr. Peter Gill of the Forensic Science Service of the Home Office said the probability that both samples contained the same DNA was "almost 99 percent." Taken in conjunction with the compelling physical skeletal evidence, the results are clear and unequivocal. Short of the Last Judgment, when the dead shall rise up and be cloaked anew with flesh, and all our doubts are scheduled to be resolved in the twinkling of an eye, we may say that the mystery of the Romanovs is solved as nearly as it is likely to be. Nevertheless we recommended in our report that the site around the pit be carefully excavated and searched for the remains of the two bodies Yurovsky said he burned. I believe such a dig might well turn up the calcined remains of Anastasia and Alexei.

"Anna Anderson" went to her grave in 1984, claiming she was Anastasia. Her body was cremated and this removed the last possibility of establishing the truth or falsity of her royal pretensions. Cremation destroys utterly all organic components of bone. No known technique can recover any DNA from cremated remains. There are supposed to be hair samples taken from Anna Anderson but these are cut hair, not rooted hair. The shafts of human hair are largely composed of dead material, devoid of significant amounts of DNA. Only hair plucked by the roots from the scalp can be tested for DNA with any real hope of success. There are some tissue samples from Anna Anderson's body, in a hospital where she underwent surgery in life. To date, legal difficulties have prevented testing these samples for their DNA.

A commission in Russia will hear our team's conclusions, and I believe the British DNA work to be the final word in resolving this old mystery. It is my understanding that the Romanov remains will be interred in St. Petersburg, which was once, briefly, known as Leningrad.

But there is one last footnote to this long, remarkable history. There is a very good possibility that the bones of the Tsar will be buried without their proper breastbone or arms! My examination of the remains convinced me that the arms and the bayonet-stabbed breastbone of Body No. 9, which has been identified as belonging to Trupp, the footman, are really those of Body No. 4, the Tsar. Body 4 was flung on top of Body 9 in the burial pit, and over the years the bones commingled closely with one another. The Russians labored valiantly to separate them, but I believe the arms and breastbone have been mixed up. I mentioned this to the Russians, and they appeared to accept my conclusion. Some of the other skeletons showed signs of mismatching and commingling as well. Unfortunately no one seems to have the authority to take the skeletons apart again and transpose the arms and breastbones to their proper owners.

It therefore seems likely that, when the last Tsar is finally entombed in St. Petersburg, he will be served in death, as he was in life, by the arms of his faithful footman.

"These Rough Notes and Our Dead Bodies . . ."

"Empty vessel, garment cast,
We that wore you long shall last.
—Another night, another day."
So my bones within me say.

Therefore they shall do my will
To-day while I am master still,
And flesh and soul, now both are strong,
Shall hale the sullen slaves along,

Before this fire of sense decay,
This smoke of thought blow clean away,
And leave with ancient night alone
The stedfast and enduring bone.

> —A. E. Housman,
> *The Immortal Part*

As I write these lines, it is a windy, bright spring day in early March in Gainesville. The live oaks have cast their leaves, and the dogwoods and azaleas are beginning to bloom. Eager young students are bicycling across campus, browsing in Goering's bookstore, studying their textbooks on sunlit lawns near dormitories.

But I am not thinking of them. I am thinking of ghosts.

I am recalling five young students, four from the University of Florida, one from nearby Santa Fe Community College, who were tortured, mutilated and murdered with demonic cruelty in August 1990. In all, the five victims suffered sixty-one stab wounds, cuts or other disfigurements. One was beheaded, and her head was placed at eye level on a bookshelf near the door of her apartment. Four of the victims were female: Sonja Larson, eighteen, of Deerfield Beach; Christi Powell, seventeen, of Jacksonville; Christa Hoyt, eighteen, of Gainesville; and Tracy Paules, twenty-three, of Miami. One was male: Manny Taboada, twenty-three, of Miami. The horror these murders aroused at the time was so keen that thousands of students literally fled Gainesville, in fear of their lives.

Today, in early March, immured in a lamplit courtroom within the Alachua County Courthouse, a jury has finished staring at pictures of these five young people, taken after their bodies were discovered. Black tape was placed over parts of the pictures considered so grisly they would have been prejudicial to the jury's reaching an impartial verdict. I can well understand these selective blackouts. In my long career I have seldom seen crime-scene photographs possessed of such sheer depravity.

In the same room with the jury, as they pondered these ghastly photographs, was the author of these terrors: the self-confessed murderer himself, Danny Harold Rolling, a drifter from Shreveport, Louisiana. Rolling claimed he was driven to kill because of abuse suffered as a child—it is a common excuse nowadays. He was arrested almost immediately on another charge after the quintuple murders (which were all committed within forty-eight hours), and only became a suspect in this case two months later, on November 2, 1990. As the prosecutor waved the horrible photographs before the jury, Rolling turned pale and appeared ill. "I've got to get out of here," he whispered at one point.

The jury was tasked with deciding his punishment: life in prison or death in the electric chair. It deliberated through one afternoon, into the evening, and reconvened the next morning, before reaching a verdict. The jury recommended death for Danny Rolling.

I remember how, in the years following his arrest, Rolling toyed with the investigators from prison, admitting nothing. He thought he had been too clever for the police. He thought he had removed all traces of his guilt from the crime scenes. He gathered up all but one piece of the duct tape he used to bind his victims. He washed two of their bodies with detergent after they were dead. He posed the bodies of the slaughtered young women in various lewd positions. Unfortunately for him, he left traces of his semen at the scene, and this identified him by means of DNA "fingerprinting."

Because of my background with weapons and wounds to bone, I was asked to be present at the autopsies, which were conducted by Dr. William Hamilton, the District 8 medical examiner. Hamilton is a quiet man of supreme competence. Unlike some of his brethren, he rigorously shuns the media limelight and works in silence. We have known each other for years, but from the first Hamilton struck me as remarkable and rare: a man who prefers to seek out the truth and to serve the people of his state with deeds of value, rather than chase the will-o'-the-wisp of fame. It is largely because of Hamilton's meticulous work that a close-meshed net of scientific evidence was drawn about Rolling. My own role in this case was minor. But I like to think that, wherever Rolling goes, I gave him one small nudge toward punishment and perdition.

My work centered around the murder weapon, and I was assisted by one of my best students, Dana Austin-Smith. Bones can reveal more about a murder weapon than skin and soft tissue, because they are not as elastic. Skin can stretch, distort, relax and finally deliquesce during decomposition. Bones, though more elastic than you might suppose, nevertheless can take and hold an impression from a murder weapon far longer, and far more accurately. By now I need not tell you that the pattern of the human skeleton is as familiar to me as the rooms of my house.

A large knife had been used in the murders. Its hilt left an imprint on one victim's back, and the point exited her chest on the opposite side, a distance of eight inches, during which the knife was fully sheathed, its entire length buried in the unfortunate girl's body.

271

But allowing for compression of the rib cage from the force and fury of the blow, the blade length might have been somewhat shorter: say seven to eight inches, to be safe.

After preparing specimens of the damaged bones, I began to examine the knife marks under a low-power stereo-microscope. I found sharp cuts from the blade, marks both sharp and dull from the back of the blade, a point mark from the knife sunk in the body of a vertebra, and an array of bone wounds that gave me the width of the blade itself, from its cutting edge to its back.

I summarized the characteristics. Length: 7–8 inches. Width: 1.25–1.5 inches. A sharp, smooth, nonserrated cutting edge. A false edge resulting from the back of the blade being sharpened behind the tip. A certain shape of hilt where the blade joined the handle. A blade whose cross-section resembled an elongated pentagon. All in all, I concluded, this was a sturdy knife, like a military weapon. It was not a thin blade like a kitchen knife. This formidable weapon had cut through thick bone without any evidence of "blade chattering," a technical term describing the distinctive cutting pattern, which a thin blade makes when it jumps slightly from side to side during use.

On the afternoon of September 7, 1990, I was at the state attorney's office in Orlando on another case. I received a telephone call, asking me to join Dr. Hamilton and the leaders of the Gainesville Homicide Task Force for a meeting. It was a fast, hundred-mile drive for me, but I arrived around 4 P.M.

We were asked about the murder weapon. Could it have been an Air Force survival knife? I said no. That knife has a sawlike, ripping design on the back of the blade, which is only five inches long—far too short to match the weapon used in these murders. Then someone asked if it might be a Marine Corps utility knife, known as a Ka-Bar. I replied that it very well might.

After the meeting I pondered the question further. I knew the general shape of the Ka-Bar but wanted to be absolutely sure. That weekend I visited a knife shop in a nearby mall, where Ka-Bars were sold. I carefully examined one, measuring it with the one-meter tape measure I always carry with me. It fit exactly the dimensions of the wounds! The clerk regarded me with some curiosity. Why, he asked finally, was I making so many measurements? I made a vague reply, but as Margaret and I were walking back to the car, I told her what I thought. The weapon used in these ghastly murders had almost certainly been a Ka-Bar.

As I have said earlier, Rolling was in custody on an unrelated charge at this point. He had not yet been focused on as a suspect in the Gainesville murders. Over three years would pass before I learned that Rolling had indeed purchased a Ka-Bar at an Army-Navy store in Tallahassee on July 17, 1990, some weeks before the killings.

The police scanned many likely areas with metal detectors, but the actual murder weapon has not surfaced to this day. On the Thursday before Rolling was scheduled to go to trial, there was a crucial evidentiary hearing, one that changed the complexion of the case completely.

State Attorney Rod Smith won the court's approval to introduce into evidence a "replica weapon," a duplicate of the lost Ka-Bar we believed had been used to commit the crimes. Not only that: the *actual skeletal remains of the victims,* taken from their bodies during the autopsies, and bearing the atrocious nicks, slashes, scorings and gougings, which the knife had caused, and which had enabled me to measure its deadly dimensions with such exactitude, were going to be allowed into evidence as well. Thus, not only the blade, but the bones themselves would be placed before the jury's gaze.

"On the Thursday prior to the beginning of the trial," a court memorandum I have before me reads, "in closed discussions before the judge, part of the discussion was about the replica knife and the accurate work which Dr. Maples had done with the knife wounds. Also discussed were the skeletal remnants . . ."

The judge ruled that all these things would be allowed into evidence. The memorandum continues:

"It was obvious that Rolling didn't want to face the photographs, let alone the remnants . . . That was the evening the defense came to Mr. Smith and offered the first of a series of plea deals."

The murderer's resolve was crumbling in the face of these fearful resurrections. The knife he imagined was hidden forever was coming back to haunt him in court. The bones of his victims were ready to return from beyond death, to rise up and smite him. The trial would begin in ninety-six hours.

Rolling quailed. On February 15, 1994, as jury selection began in his trial, the accused man suddenly pleaded guilty to five counts of murder and three counts of rape.

"I've been running all my life," he declared. "And there are some things you can't run from anymore."

There began the punishment phase of the case, during which the jury had to decide whether Rolling deserved the death penalty or life in prison. Prosecutor Smith showed the jurors the replica knife, the twin of the Ka-Bar I had identified as the murder weapon. The bones were mercifully withheld from the jurors' sight. The dark blade danced back and forth before their eyes. Together with the hood Rolling wore, and the photographs of his victims, the knife must have made an overwhelming impression on the panel. Their verdict: Death. Rolling received five death sentences from Judge Stan Morris.

"Five years! You're going to go down in five years! You understand that? In less than five years!" screamed Mario Taboada, the brother of the slain Manuel Taboada. He was predicting that Rolling would exhaust all his appeals and be executed by 1999. The judge ordered Taboada ejected from the courtroom. Gradually the din subsided. One of the darkest chapters in Gainesville's history was closed.

All in all, the Rolling case was a significant victory for the science of forensic anthropology in Florida, one that saved the taxpayer the immense cost of a full-blown trial, and the victims' relatives the terrible pain of hearing in a public courtroom exactly how these innocent young people had died. It remains one of the most extraordinary cases in my experience, one that amply demonstrated the sheer power possessed by human bones: the power to bear witness to the truth beyond death; the power to avenge the innocent; the power to terrify the guilty.

Today, at the side of 34th Street in Gainesville, near the crest of a hill, there is a brilliantly painted section of wall dedicated to student graffiti and free speech. Everyone in Gainesville knows it simply as "The Wall." It runs beneath a fence draped with kudzu vine at the boundary of the campus golf course, and its shape rather reminds you of a railroad cutting, revealing all sorts of multicolored minerals, some of them precious, some of them fool's gold.

Anyone is welcome to paint a message on this wall, which is by now a local landmark and a University of Florida tradition. Most of the messages are cheery, or silly, or affectionate, or whimsical. But amid the valentines, the happy birthday wishes and the pleas to save the rain forest is a single dark panel in the wall at the very top of the hill. It contains the names of the five murder victims, neatly lettered against a black background, accompanied by the single word: RE-MEMBER. If this panel fades or is accidentally defaced, someone always renews it and repaints the names. I pass it twice a day, and I do indeed remember.

I have purposely kept this account of the Gainesville murders for last, not because they struck so close to home—Rolling could have killed anywhere, in any town—but because I believe there is a moral to this melancholy tale. It is simply that the lamp of science, properly grasped and directed, can shine its rays into the very heart of darkness. It can seek out and snare the most artful evildoer in a bright, unequivocal beam of truth. It cannot raise the dead, but it can make them speak, accuse and identify the agent of death. With the capture and punishment of the criminal responsible, the families and relatives of those slain can win a small measure of peace amid their infinite sorrow. With each solved case, with every confession, we extend our knowledge of the criminal mind and its methods, and we render the threat of capture and punishment all the more real and credible.

Yet as I look back on my life, and ahead to the future, I am given pause by the vast amount of work that still needs to be done. Mine is a small field, and it is always going to be a small field; but there is no excuse for its being as small as it is today. Cases now throng in daily to the C. A. Pound Human Identification Laboratory, in such jostling multitudes that I cannot address them all and must focus only on the most serious ones. When the telephone rings, my heartbeat quickens. I know that it is most likely the police, and I know what they will say, for I have heard it hundreds of times now:

"Doc, we've got a problem . . ."

And the problem is always a body, or what is left of one. They tell me they've set up security around the remains. They tell me police officers are guarding and preserving the scene. They ask: can I come immediately? Because I no longer have an undergraduate class load, I am able to break free more often than not. If I am rescued by a murder from a dull and dismal faculty meeting, so much the better! In the case of the three shotgunned drug dealers found in a pit near La Belle, I enlisted the aid of an archaeologist colleague and we both managed to be in Fort Myers, 230 miles away, by dark. By 8 A.M. the next morning we were in the death pit, hard at work.

With crime moving to the forefront of the American domestic political agenda, it would appear likely that investigators such as myself can look forward to busy years and full employment. But against this must be weighed the fact that few universities are willing to underwrite programs like mine, which combine pure academic research with applications in the "real world," and the fact that few state law enforcement agencies have the money or inclination to avail themselves of the services of a trained forensic anthropologist.

So we fall between two stools. We are regarded by our fellow academics almost as common laborers with dirty hands, who traffic in mundane, workaday police matters, instead of devoting ourselves to pure research. On the other hand the police tend to regard us as woolgatherers and cloud-dwellers from the ivory tower, with no experience of the dark side of life. When I am visiting a new law enforcement agency for the first time, I often assume the persona of the innocent, fuddy-duddy professor who has to have everything pointed out to him. This role-playing won't win me any Oscars, but it humors the police, does no harm and gets results far more quickly than would an attitude of haughty, know-it-all, intellectual arrogance.

Yet sometimes I am prey to doubts. Who will replace me, and others like me? Who will hire the students I train? I cannot say. The need is there. It cries out to heaven. As I compose these lines, there are forty-eight charred corpses left over from the fiery explosion at the Branch Davidian compound outside Waco, awaiting identification. My colleague, Clyde Snow, is in Chiapas, Mexico, looking at the bodies of slain Zapatista revolutionaries, to see if they were murdered by the Mexican army after they surrendered. Remains of MIAs from the Korean War are being returned to America, and their names are a riddle as yet unsolved. The mass graves in Bosnia shout to the skies for discovery and vengeance. Yet programs in forensic anthropology languish, and well-trained young scholars go begging for work.

In my lifetime I have seen programs rise and fall like shooting stars. Once upon a time, at the University of Kansas, three of the gods of forensic anthropology—Tom McKern, Ellis Kerley and Bill Bass—were all on the faculty *at the same time.* They attracted and taught scores of students, many of whom are among the leading people in our field today. Then, almost overnight, they were scattered to the four winds. Bass left one year, McKern and Kerley the next. The university hired a human geneticist, rather than anyone in bone. The same melancholy story is about to be repeated at the University of Arizona, where Walt Birkby has built up a fantastic program. Birkby's students are probably the best-trained of any in the United States. But Walt is retiring in a couple of years, and the university has already announced he will not be replaced. Therefore he has closed admission to his program. He takes no new students.

Bill Bass has just retired from Tennessee. The university is going to replace him with an assistant professor, but without Bill's active guidance that program will undoubtedly change. I will retire myself in a few years and, even though University of Florida President John Lombardi has worked miracles in other areas, I seriously doubt whether the C. A. Pound Human Identification Laboratory will survive my departure.

If these memoirs have demonstrated anything, I would hope that it is that forensic anthropology is a discipline useful to society. Had I the power to command it, I should decree that each state have at least one forensic anthropologist working in its crime laboratory. Climate and crime rates have to be taken into consideration of course. A forensic anthropologist would probably starve to death in a cold state like Maine or Minnesota—bodies last forever in those arctic regions! He might find little to do in a state like New Hampshire, where there are only a couple of dozen murders in a year. But here in the sunny, homicidal South there are plenty of bodies to go around, and plenty of bugs to feast on them. Decomposition is swift and sure, and nameless skeletons accumulate in thousands, each beseeching us silently for identification.

Larger states, such as Texas, California, New York, Florida and the like, could easily employ several scientists like me, and none would be idle, I assure you. I know from long experience that I can't begin to look at all the cases demanding my attention in the state of Florida. A handful of states, those having a single medical examiner with statewide responsibility, have appointed forensic anthropologists to that office, but they are few and far between. As our elected officials bay like bloodhounds over the crime issue, as our state budgets allocate large sums for prisons, police training and equipment, parole officers, boot camps for teenagers and heaven knows what else, they overlook utterly the need to fund research by universities to develop new scientific techniques necessary to apprehend criminals. The Forensic Sciences Foundation has started a small grant program to provide funds, largely supported by donations from members of the American Academy of Forensic Scientists. But none of us is a Croesus or a Rockefeller. Our little fund is growing painfully slowly. It can only provide a few modest grants each year.

Seldom does a week go by without my receiving a visit or a telephone call from some young person eager to go into forensic anthropology. Will I accept him or her as a student? Alas, I don't have the money to support large numbers of students, nor the space in which to teach and train them, nor the time to give them all the attention they deserve. Even if I were to take them in, where would they go when they left me, having won their doctorates? Where would they get jobs? No doubt a handful of them would, as I did, work their way into a university system and slowly establish a practice. Most wouldn't. That is the bitter truth.

The murder and suicide rate in the state of Florida could easily furnish cases for six full-time forensic anthropologists. In my daydreams I locate them on a mind-map of the state with stickpins: there would be one in the Panhandle, another in Gainesville, another in Orlando, one in southwest Florida and one, perhaps two, in Miami. Miami, as we all know, is a very special place: the deadliest city in the most crime-ridden state in the Union. Forensic anthropologists would find plenty to do there. They would be useful to state medical examiners in skeletonized cases, cases involving burn victims, decomposed bodies and the like. We could even help identify fresh bodies belonging to the nameless and the homeless, who are flocking to Florida—and to Florida's morgues—in ever increasing numbers nowadays. Some medical examiners' offices perform over three thousand autopsies each year.

I can't be everywhere. I have been under as many as four separate subpoenas, to testify in four separate cities, all on the same day. One prosecutor, jokingly I hope, actually threatened to throw me in jail if I did not testify for him, rather than in another case scheduled for that day! Ours is a very large state. If a decomposed body is found in the Florida Keys, there is no way I can be on the scene immediately. Sometimes the remains are shipped to me, if I cannot go to them. Federal Express won't transport human remains, including cremains, but the U. S. Post Office has no such qualms, as long as the remains are identified as "evidence" or "specimens." But if we had a forensic anthropologist stationed in Miami, these cases could be attended to on the spot.

Such are the thoughts that sometimes visit me at night. But "sufficient unto the day is the evil thereof," as the Bible says. Whenever I am beset by doubts over the future of my discipline, or the career opportunities for my students, or the fate of my laboratory after I am gone, I look at the filing cabinets filled with case reports. Here at least is solid, measurable progress. Here I can claim to have made a difference.

In days when people knew more Latin than they do now, someone composed a deeply moving inscription that can still be read over the lintel of the New York City medical examiner's office:

Taceant Colloquia. Effugiat Risus. Hic Locus Est Ubi Mors Gaudet Succurrere Vitae.

[Let idle talk be silenced. Let laughter be banished. Here is the place where Death delights to succour Life.]

I have no room over my laboratory door lintel for an engraved inscription, but if I did I would choose the last words of the explorer, Robert Falcon Scott, who perished in the frozen wastes of Antarctica in 1912, of hunger and exposure, in a place that was only a few miles from food and safety. The last entry in his diary read:

Had we lived, I should have had a tale to tell of the hardihood, endurance and courage of my companions, that would have stirred the heart of every Englishman. These rough notes and our dead bodies must tell the tale.

That's how I feel about the skeletons here in my laboratory. They have tales to tell us, even though they are dead. It is up to me, the forensic anthropologist, to catch their mute cries and whispers, and to interpret them for the living, as long as I am able.

Acknowledgments

This book could not have been written, and the life it describes could not have been lived, were it not for my wife, Margaret Kelley. Margaret and I are old comrades now. We met in Miss Berry's Spanish class in my sophomore year at North Dallas High School. At the end of the year Miss Berry struck a deal with me: she'd give me a C if I would promise never to take Spanish again. I readily agreed. I never mastered the language of Cervantes and Calderón, but I won Margaret.

We married in 1958 and through all these years she has been the spark that has galvanized me to greater effort. It was she who persuaded me to accept a job offer to work with baboons in Africa, and take her with me, even though she was five months pregnant. Both of our children, Lisa and Cynthia, were born in Africa. She has always been the more energetic and adventuresome of us two, and her courage and patience with the outlandish side of my work has always amazed me. There is certainly no one more skilled and experienced than she is, when it comes to removing bloodstains from laundry! Nor are there many wives who could sit unflinchingly through a slide presentation of time-lapsed photography depicting the action of maggots on the human face, as Margaret once did at a convention of the American Academy of Forensic Scientists. Her clarity of intellect and strong heart have upborne me all my adult life. Without her I might have been a mere, dull measurer of bones. With her, I have never become unmoored from the lively touch of humanity.

Acknowledgments

My professional indebtedness to my old teacher, Tom McKern, and to my colleagues, old and young, such as Clyde Snow, Michael Baden, Lowell Levine, Doug Ubelaker, as well as to William Hamilton, the District 8 chief medical examiner, has already been hinted at in these pages, but I would like to re-echo it here. Without the support of the Florida medical examiners, especially Wallace Graves and Joe Davis, my story would have been sparse indeed. Special mention must be made of Curtis Mertz, of Ashtabula, Ohio, who helped me solve the puzzling Meek-Jennings case described in Chapter 11. Mertz assembled all the dental information, the postmortem remains, and the antemortem radiographs in this labyrinthine affair. We worked very much as a team, and the final, conclusive dental identifications are owed to his keen eye.

I owe special debts to Bob Benfer, who got me started on historical cases; to Bill Goza, expeditor and amazing resource; and to the Wentworth Foundation. The administration of the University of Florida is gratefully acknowledged.

C. Addison Pound, Jr., benefactor of the laboratory bearing his name and that of his parents, has given me the freedom to develop my interests. His continued support of the goals of this laboratory is a shining example of how a private citizen can have an impact on crime and assisting its victims.

Margaret's help was invaluable to me in reading the manuscript and making many useful suggestions. She took several of the photographs that appear in this book, and helped me assemble the rest. I would like to acknowledge the assistance of Yale's Beinecke Library for a photograph of Tsar Nicholas's daughters and for access to other photographic archives. I am grateful for the help and hospitality of Dr. Alexander Avdonin, who enabled us to view and analyze the skeletons of the Tsar and his family. An earlier, shorter version of the account of the Ekaterinburg skeletons appeared in the *Miami Herald*'s *Tropic* magazine, and permission to reuse this material is herewith gratefully acknowledged. Our literary agent, Esther Newberg, surpassed Rumpelstiltskin in spinning gold from raw flax. Our editors at Doubleday, Bill Thomas and Rob Robertson, were enthusiastic, Argus-eyed and patient, at all the right times.

William R. Maples, Ph.D.

Michael C. Browning

Index

Index

Index